MAHA

A Blueprint for a Thriving Nation

Make America Healthy Again

MAHA

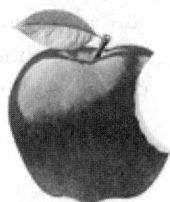

A Blueprint for a Thriving Nation

CHAUNCEY CRANDALL, M.D.

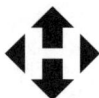

Humanix Books
www.humanixbooks.com

Humanix Books
MAHA: Make America Healthy Again

Humanix Books, P.O. Box 20989, West Palm Beach, FL 33416, USA
www.humanixbooks.com | info@humanixbooks.com

Disclaimer: The information presented in this book is not specific medical advice for any individual and should not substitute medical advice from a health professional. If you have (or think you may have) a medical problem, speak to your doctor or a health professional immediately about your risk and possible treatments. Do not engage in any care or treatment without consulting a medical professional.

Humanix Books titles may be purchased for educational, business, or sales promotional use. For information about special discounts for bulk purchases, please contact the Special Markets Department at info@ humanixbooks.com.

Cover, et. al.: Apple: iStock/Marat Musabirov
Dr. Crandall: Staff Photographer

Cover Design: Ben Davis

ISBN: 978-163006-314-6 (Hardcover)
ISBN: 978-163006-315-3 (E-book)

Printed in the United States of America
10 9 8 7 6 5 4 3 2 1

To my wife, Deborah, my sons, Christian and Chad,
and the patients the Lord has entrusted to my care.

All to the glory of God.

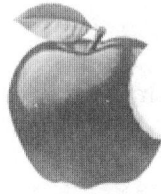

CONTENTS

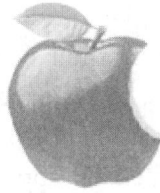

A DOCTOR'S PRESCRIPTION FOR AMERICA

've dedicated my entire career to understanding the complexities of health—from the deep-rooted cultural influences I studied as an anthropologist to the cutting-edge medical treatments I've delivered as a cardiologist and preventive medicine physician. The path I've traveled has been anything but conventional, but it's this breadth of experience that gives me a unique perspective on the current health crisis facing America. As I've seen firsthand, the state of our nation's health is at a critical tipping point, and it's time we take a bold, informed approach to turn things around.

Early in my career, my work as a medical anthropologist took me to remote parts of the world, where I studied traditional healing practices and the profound impact of culture on health. It was there, in villages far removed from modern medicine, that I began to see the powerful role lifestyle and environment play in shaping our well-being. This understanding became the bedrock of my approach to medicine: Health is not just the absence of disease—it's the result of our daily choices, our environment, and our cultural practices.

When I moved into the field of cardiology and preventive medicine, I brought this holistic perspective with me. I've spent decades on the frontlines, treating patients with severe heart disease, many of whom were given little hope. Yet, I've seen miraculous recoveries—patients reversing their conditions through targeted, lifestyle-based interventions. These experiences have solidified my belief that much of what ails us can be prevented, managed, or even reversed if we take a comprehensive approach that addresses the root causes, not just the symptoms.

But my work hasn't been confined within the walls of a hospital. As a medical missionary, I've traveled to some of the poorest, most underserved regions of the world. In these challenging environments, I've delivered life-saving care and witnessed the incredible resilience of people when given the right support and resources. These missions have taught me that the principles of preventive health and holistic care are universal—they work whether I'm treating a heart patient in Palm Beach or a child with an infection in rural Haiti.

In this book, I bring together everything I've learned from my diverse career. I tackle the most pressing health issues of our time, from poor diet and lack of exercise to the mental health crisis and the controversial topic of vaccine safety. I don't shy away from difficult conversations. Instead, I address them head-on, with a commitment to honesty, transparency, and patient advocacy. I lay out a clear, actionable plan for how each of us can take control of our own health, and how our communities and government can support a healthier society.

"Make America Healthy Again" is not just a call to action—it's a comprehensive guide rooted in decades of clinical practice, academic research, and real-world experience. I've seen what works and what doesn't. I've seen patients transform their lives and reclaim their health. And I've seen entire communities rise up to tackle health disparities and make lasting changes.

This book is my vision for a healthier America, based on proven strategies and a lifetime of learning. It's about creating a culture of health, one that values prevention, embraces holistic care, and prioritizes equity. Together, we can build a nation where everyone has the opportunity to live a long, vibrant, and healthy life. I'm here to guide you on that journey, drawing on everything I've learned along the way. Let's get started. Let's Make America Healthy Again!

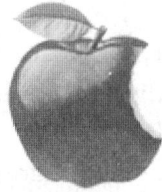

CHAPTER ONE

THE HEALTH CRISIS IN AMERICA

The United States is facing a growing and complex health crisis that threatens not only the well-being of individuals but also the stability of the healthcare system and the nation's economic future. Obesity rates are at an all-time high, chronic diseases such as heart disease and diabetes continue to rise, mental health issues are escalating, and addiction has reached epidemic proportions. These health challenges are intertwined with lifestyle choices, environmental factors, and socio-economic inequalities. The question is no longer whether America is unhealthy, but rather how we can reverse this alarming trend and restore public health to the forefront of national priorities.

THE OBESITY EPIDEMIC

One of the most visible signs of the health crisis in America is the soaring rate of obesity. According to the Centers for Disease Control and Prevention (CDC), more than 42% of adults and nearly 20% of children in the United States are classified as obese, a significant increase over the past few decades. Obesity is not merely an issue of appearance; it is a major risk factor for a wide range of health problems, including heart disease, stroke, type 2 diabetes, certain cancers, and premature death.

The roots of the obesity epidemic are deep and multifaceted. The rise of ultra-processed and fast foods—high in sugar, unhealthy fats, and empty calories—has contributed significantly to poor dietary habits. Busy lifestyles, particularly in urban areas, have led many Americans to rely on quick, cheap, and highly caloric meals. At the same time, physical activity levels have plummeted due to sedentary work environments, increased screen time, and urban designs that discourage walking or biking.

In many cases, individuals face limited access to healthy foods, especially in low-income and rural areas, where grocery stores are scarce, and fresh produce is expensive. These areas, known as "food deserts," make it difficult for people to maintain a healthy diet, further exacerbating the obesity problem. Additionally, the food industry's aggressive marketing of sugary drinks, snacks, and fast foods to children and adolescents has fostered unhealthy eating habits from an early age.

CHRONIC DISEASES ON THE RISE

Chronic diseases are responsible for 70% of all deaths in the United States and are the leading drivers of the nation's $3.8 trillion in annual healthcare costs. Conditions such as heart disease, cancer, diabetes, and respiratory diseases are not only preventable in many cases but also deeply rooted in the same factors driving the obesity crisis. Poor diet, lack of physical activity, tobacco use, and excessive alcohol consumption are the primary contributors to these diseases.

Heart disease remains the leading cause of death in America, accounting for approximately 697,000 deaths each year. It is often linked to high blood pressure, high cholesterol, and obesity, all of which are preventable through lifestyle changes. Similarly, type 2 diabetes, which affects more than 34 million Americans, is closely tied to obesity and sedentary behavior. The rise in diabetes cases has also led to an increase in related complications, such as kidney failure, blindness, and amputations.

Cancer, the second leading cause of death in the United States today, is another chronic disease influenced by lifestyle and environmental factors. While some cancers are genetic, many are linked to smoking, poor diet, alcohol use, and exposure to toxins. Lung cancer, for example, is still the deadliest cancer in the United States, largely due to tobacco use, while colorectal cancer has been tied to poor diet and low fiber intake.

THE MENTAL HEALTH CRISIS

In recent years, the mental health crisis in America has become more visible and more urgent. Anxiety, depression, and suicide rates are at historic highs, with the COVID-19 pandemic further exacerbating mental health issues. According to the National Institute of Mental Health, nearly one in five U.S. adults lives with a mental illness, and rates of mental health disorders have been rising steadily among teenagers and young adults.

Stress, loneliness, and burnout have become common features of modern American life, with the pressures of work, social media, and economic instability taking a toll on mental well-being. The stigma surrounding mental illness, coupled with inadequate access to mental health services, especially in underserved communities, has left many Americans suffering in silence. Even those who seek help often face barriers such as long wait times for therapy, high costs, or insufficient insurance coverage.

The rise in mental health disorders has also contributed to the opioid crisis and substance abuse epidemic, with many people turning to drugs and alcohol as a way to cope with stress, trauma, or untreated mental illness. The opioid epidemic alone has claimed the lives of over 500,000 Americans since 1999, with overdose deaths continuing to rise due to the increased availability of synthetic opioids like fentanyl.

ECONOMIC AND SOCIETAL COSTS

The health crisis in America is not just a personal or medical issue; it is an economic and societal burden. The healthcare system is strained under the weight of treating preventable diseases, with chronic conditions accounting for 90% of the nation's healthcare expenditures. The costs of treating obesity-related illnesses, managing diabetes, and addressing the complications of heart disease and cancer are staggering. Furthermore, the loss of productivity due to illness, absenteeism, and premature death has significant economic repercussions.

In addition to the direct medical costs, the societal costs of poor health are profound. Families are often financially devastated by medical bills, especially in a country where medical bankruptcy is common. Communities are fractured by the tolls of addiction, mental illness, and chronic disease. The workforce suffers as more people become too sick to work, and the educational system struggles to address the health needs of children who are growing up in environments that do not support healthy habits.

Moreover, health disparities across racial, ethnic, and socioeconomic lines deepen the divide between rich and poor, healthy and sick. African Americans, Hispanic Americans, and Native Americans face higher rates of chronic disease and lower life expectancy due to systemic barriers to healthcare, nutritious food, and safe environments for exercise. These disparities are not only unjust but also costly, as they contribute to the overall burden on the healthcare system.

ENVIRONMENTAL AND LIFESTYLE FACTORS

The health crisis in America cannot be fully understood without considering the broader environmental and lifestyle factors at play. Urbanization, industrialization, and technological advances have transformed the way Americans live, often to the detriment of their health. Cities are designed with cars in mind, not pedestrians, leading to fewer opportunities for physical activity. Air pollution, especially in industrial areas, contributes to respiratory problems and exacerbates conditions like asthma.

At the same time, technology has made daily life more sedentary. The average American spends hours each day sitting—whether at a desk, in a car, or in front of a screen. This lack of movement, coupled with high-calorie diets, has created a perfect storm for weight gain and related health problems. Moreover, the rise of social media and digital devices has been linked to mental health issues such as anxiety, depression, and sleep disorders, particularly among young people.

THE ROLE OF POLICY AND PREVENTION

Addressing America's health crisis requires a paradigm shift from treating diseases to preventing them. The healthcare system has long been reactive, focusing on managing symptoms rather than addressing the root causes of illness. However, prevention is not only more effective but also more cost-efficient. Encouraging healthy eating, regular physical activity, and mental well-being could dramatically reduce the burden of chronic diseases.

Public policy plays a crucial role in shaping health outcomes. For instance, taxation on sugary beverages has been shown to reduce consumption and can be used to fund public health programs. Similarly, stricter regulations on food labeling and advertising, particularly to children, could help combat the obesity epidemic. Urban planning that prioritizes green spaces, bike lanes, and pedestrian-friendly streets would encourage physical activity and improve overall health.

Education is also key. Schools can play a central role in teaching children healthy habits from a young age, and public health campaigns can raise awareness about the importance of diet, exercise, and mental health. In addition, improving access to healthcare, particularly preventive services, can help catch health problems early and reduce the long-term costs of treatment.

HOPE AND A PATH FORWARD

The health crisis in America is a complex and multifaceted issue that requires a coordinated and comprehensive response. It is not enough to treat the symptoms of obesity, chronic disease, mental illness, and addiction; we must address the root causes. This includes reforming the food system, promoting physical activity, improving access to mental health services, and enacting policies that support healthy living.

By shifting the focus from treatment to prevention, America can begin to reverse the trends that have led to its current health crisis. It will require the collaboration of individuals, communities, healthcare providers, policymakers, and businesses to make America healthy again. The benefits of such a shift will not only be seen in improved health outcomes but also in a stronger economy, a more vibrant society, and a better quality of life for all Americans.

DR. CRANDALL'S AMERICA:
A Reflection on the Health Crisis

As a physician with decades of experience in cardiology and preventive medicine, I've witnessed firsthand the evolution of health in America—and not all of it has been for the better. The patients I've treated and the stories I've encountered are both a testament to the resilience of the human spirit and a stark reminder of the systemic issues that continue to plague our healthcare system.

One patient I'll never forget was a man in his mid-fifties who came to me with severe heart disease. He had been living with uncontrolled diabetes for years, a condition that had silently damaged his body. When we discussed his history, it became clear that much of this could have been prevented. His diet was a typical reflection of the Standard American Diet (SAD)—high in processed foods and sugars, low in fresh produce—and his physical activity had been limited due to long work hours and financial stress. He told me, "Doctor, no one ever told me I could change this. I thought it was just my fate." After months of hard work together—addressing his diet, starting an exercise routine, and managing his stress—he began to regain control of his health. But I couldn't help but wonder how many others like him never get that chance.

Unfortunately, not all stories have such a hopeful outcome. Over the years, I've treated countless patients who came to me too late—when the damage from chronic conditions like diabetes, hypertension, or obesity was irreversible. I've seen young people in their twenties suffer from diseases that were once considered rare at their age, such as heart attacks or severe metabolic disorders. What's most alarming is the trend: these issues are becoming more common, not less.

One striking example was a young mother of two who arrived in the emergency room with a heart attack. She was 35 years old, working two jobs, and barely had time to care for herself. When I asked about her lifestyle, she admitted she relied on fast food because it was cheap and quick, and she hadn't seen a doctor in years because she couldn't afford regular check-ups. Stories like hers highlight the devastating intersection of economic challenges, lack of access to healthcare, and the growing prevalence of chronic diseases in America.

Yet, amid these challenges, there are glimmers of progress. I've seen patients and communities rally together to adopt healthier lifestyles. For example, in one rural community I worked with, a local church began offering free weekly fitness classes and nutrition workshops, transforming the lives of many in the congregation. These grassroots efforts remind me that change is possible, even in the face of overwhelming odds.

But the bigger picture remains troubling. As a doctor, I often feel like I'm putting out fires rather than preventing them. The healthcare system is largely reactive, focusing on treating illnesses rather than preventing them. Patients often come to me after years of neglecting their health—sometimes because they didn't know better, but often because the system failed them. Preventive care isn't prioritized, access to healthy food is limited in many communities, and the stress of modern life continues to erode mental and physical health.

What's clear to me is that the American health crisis isn't just about individual choices—it's about a system that makes those choices harder. From the food industry's relentless push of unhealthy products to the barriers that keep people from accessing affordable care, the deck is stacked against too many Americans. Yet, I remain hopeful. With the right policies, education, and community support, we can begin to reverse these trends. But it will take a collective effort, one that starts with acknowledging the depth of the problem and committing to real, systemic change.

These stories, and the lessons they've taught me, fuel my determination to advocate for a healthier America. Each patient I've treated has shown me the power of resilience and the potential for transformation when given the right tools and support. It's my hope that by addressing these issues head-on, we can create a healthcare system— and a society—that prioritizes prevention, compassion, and equity for all.

R℞ Dr. Crandall's Prescription for the Health Crisis in America

✔ **Take Ownership of Your Health.** Recognize the role of personal responsibility in improving health outcomes. Commit to making small, consistent changes in diet, exercise, and lifestyle to prevent chronic illnesses.

✔ **Prioritize Preventive Care.** Schedule regular check-ups and screenings to catch potential health issues early. Stay informed about vaccinations and preventive measures relevant to your age and risk factors.

✔ **Acknowledge the Role of Lifestyle Choices.** Understand how everyday habits, such as sedentary behavior, poor diet, and inadequate sleep, contribute to chronic disease. Begin addressing these habits one step at a time.

✔ **Stay Educated About Health Risks.** Learn about the common health challenges Americans face, such as obesity, diabetes, and heart disease, and the specific steps you can take to mitigate your risks.

✔ **Engage in Community Health Resources.** Leverage local health programs, fitness classes, or wellness events to stay active and connected with others who share similar goals.

✔ **Focus on Stress Management.** Incorporate mindfulness practices, such as meditation, deep breathing, or yoga, to address stress, which is a significant contributor to poor health outcomes.

✔ **Set Realistic and Achievable Goals.** Start with attainable goals, like walking 10 minutes daily or reducing sugar intake, to build confidence and momentum toward larger health improvements.

Resources

Healthcare.gov
The official government healthcare site for health insurance marketplace plans, subsidies, and enrollment.

Medicare.gov
Information on Medicare eligibility, plans, and coverage for seniors and for people with certain disabilities.

Kaiser Family Foundation
Provides research and comparisons of health insurance plans, coverage options, and policy updates (https://www.kff.org).

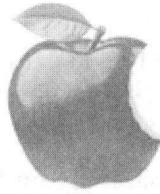

CHAPTER TWO

FOOD AS MEDICINE

I n recent years, the concept of "food as medicine" has gained increasing attention as a vital approach to improving health and preventing chronic diseases. The old adage "You are what you eat" carries more truth than ever, as a growing body of scientific evidence links diet with the prevention and management of a wide range of conditions, from heart disease and diabetes to cancer and mental health issues. In contrast, the Standard American Diet (SAD), characterized by highly processed foods, excessive sugars, and unhealthy fats, is fueling a health crisis that threatens the well-being of millions of Americans.

The philosophy behind food as medicine is simple: What we eat can either harm or heal us. Nutrient-rich, whole foods support the body's natural defenses, promote optimal health, and even reverse disease. Conversely, a poor diet contributes to inflammation, oxidative stress, and a weakened immune system, all of which are underlying factors in chronic disease. In this chapter, we explore how food can serve as medicine, the dangers of the SAD diet, and how shifting our approach to nutrition can revolutionize public health.

THE POWER OF NUTRITION IN PREVENTING AND REVERSING DISEASE

Nutrition plays a critical role in every function of the body, from energy production and immune function to mental clarity and mood regulation. Yet, the significance of food as a tool for health is often overlooked in favor of pharmaceutical interventions. While medications certainly have their place, particularly in acute or advanced illness, they often come with side effects and do little to address the root causes of disease. Food, on the other hand, offers a natural and accessible way to support the body's healing processes.

Consider cardiovascular disease, the leading cause of death in the United States. Decades of research have shown that a diet rich in whole grains, fruits, vegetables, nuts, seeds, and healthy fats like olive oil can significantly reduce the risk of heart disease. The Mediterranean diet, in particular, has been praised for its heart-protective effects, lowering the risk of heart attacks and strokes by as much as 30%. This diet emphasizes plant-based foods, lean proteins like fish, and healthy fats, while minimizing red meat, processed foods, and refined sugars.

Similarly, type 2 diabetes—a condition closely linked to poor diet and obesity—can often be prevented and even reversed through dietary changes. Studies have shown that individuals who adopt a plant-based diet, rich in fiber, complex carbohydrates, and healthy fats, can improve insulin sensitivity, reduce blood sugar levels, and lose weight, all of which contribute to diabetes remission. In fact, research from institutions like Harvard University has demonstrated that a diet centered around whole, minimally processed foods can reduce the risk of developing diabetes by up to 80%.

Cancer, another leading cause of death, is also deeply influenced by diet. While no single food can prevent cancer, a diet rich in antioxidants, phytonutrients, and anti-inflammatory compounds has been shown to reduce the risk of certain types of cancer, particularly those linked to lifestyle factors. Cruciferous vegetables like broccoli, kale, and Brussels sprouts contain compounds that have been shown to inhibit cancer cell growth. Likewise, foods like berries, garlic, turmeric, and green tea possess powerful anti-inflammatory and antioxidant properties that support the body's defense against oxidative stress and chronic inflammation, both of which play a role in cancer development.

THE STANDARD AMERICAN DIET AND ITS HEALTH CONSEQUENCES

Despite the growing understanding of the benefits of a whole-foods, plant-based diet, the Standard American Diet remains heavily reliant on processed and convenience foods. The typical American diet is high in saturated and trans fats, added sugars, and sodium, while being low in fiber, vitamins, and minerals. These dietary patterns are fueling an epidemic of obesity, heart disease, diabetes, and other chronic illnesses.

One of the most harmful aspects of the SAD is its over-reliance on processed foods. Processed foods are often stripped of their natural nutrients during manufacturing, leaving behind empty calories that contribute to weight gain and poor health. For example, refined grains like white bread and pasta are missing the fiber and nutrients found in whole grains, making them rapidly digestible and prone to causing blood sugar spikes. Similarly, processed meats like bacon, sausage, and hot dogs have been linked to an increased risk of colorectal cancer, heart disease, and other health issues due to their high levels of saturated fats, sodium, and preservatives.

Added sugars are another major culprit in the SAD. The average American consumes about 17 teaspoons of added sugar per day, far exceeding the recommended limit of 6 teaspoons for women and 9 teaspoons for men. Sugary drinks, snacks, and desserts are the primary sources of these excess sugars, which contribute to weight gain, insulin resistance, and increased risk of type 2 diabetes. Sugary beverages, in particular, are a leading driver of obesity in both children and adults. When consumed in excess, they provide little nutritional value and lead to overeating, as liquid calories do not trigger the same sense of fullness as solid foods.

Unhealthy fats, such as trans fats and excessive saturated fats, also feature prominently in the SAD. These fats are commonly found in fried foods, fast foods, baked goods, and packaged snacks. Trans fats, in particular, have been banned in many countries due to their strong association with heart disease, yet they persist in some processed foods in the United States. Meanwhile, diets high in saturated fats—primarily from red meat and dairy products—are linked to higher levels of LDL (bad) cholesterol, which increases the risk of heart disease.

THE ROLE OF FOOD POLICY IN PUBLIC HEALTH

Food policy plays a significant role in shaping the dietary habits of Americans. Government subsidies for crops like corn, soy, and wheat have made processed foods cheap and widely available, while fruits, vegetables, and other whole foods remain more expensive in comparison. This has created an environment in which unhealthy food is often more affordable and accessible than healthy alternatives, particularly in low-income communities.

The food industry also heavily influences public perception and consumption through advertising and marketing, especially targeting children and adolescents. Billions of dollars are spent each year promoting sugary cereals, snacks, fast foods, and sugary drinks to young audiences, shaping their preferences and behaviors from an early age. This has contributed to the normalization of unhealthy eating patterns and has made it more challenging for parents to encourage healthier choices.

Reforming food policy is crucial to making healthy food more accessible and affordable for all Americans. Policies that incentivize the production and consumption of fruits, vegetables, whole grains, and plant-based proteins could help shift the national diet away from processed foods and toward a more nutritious, sustainable model. Taxing sugary drinks, as has been done in cities like Philadelphia and Berkeley, has been shown to reduce consumption and generate revenue for public health initiatives. Similarly, improving food labeling and restricting the marketing of unhealthy foods to children could help consumers make more informed choices and reduce the prevalence of diet-related diseases.

FOOD DESERTS AND FOOD INSECURITY

Food deserts—areas where access to fresh, healthy, and affordable food is limited—are a major barrier to healthy eating in many parts of the United States. These areas, often found in low-income urban and rural communities, lack supermarkets or grocery stores that carry fresh produce, whole grains, and other nutritious options. Instead, residents of food deserts may rely on convenience stores or fast food outlets, which primarily offer processed and unhealthy foods.

Food insecurity, or the lack of consistent access to enough food for an active, healthy life, is another critical issue affecting millions of Americans. According to the U.S. Department of Agriculture (USDA), over 38 million Americans, including 12 million children, lived in food-insecure households in 2020. Food insecurity is closely linked to poor diet quality, as individuals facing economic hardship often prioritize cheap, calorie-dense foods over nutrient-rich options. This pattern contributes to higher rates of obesity and chronic disease among food-insecure populations.

Addressing food deserts and food insecurity requires targeted interventions at the community and policy levels. Expanding programs like the Supplemental Nutrition Assistance Program (SNAP) to provide greater access to fresh fruits and vegetables, supporting farmers' markets in underserved areas, and encouraging the development of grocery stores in food deserts are all potential solutions. Additionally, initiatives that promote urban gardening and local food production can help empower communities to grow their own food and improve self-sufficiency.

THE FUTURE OF FOOD AS MEDICINE

As the evidence continues to mount in favor of food as medicine, a growing movement is pushing for a more integrated approach to healthcare that emphasizes nutrition as a cornerstone of disease prevention and treatment. Healthcare systems are beginning to recognize the value of prescribing not just medications but also dietary changes to improve patient outcomes. Programs like "food pharmacies," where patients can receive free or discounted healthy foods alongside nutritional counseling, are gaining traction in hospitals and clinics across the country.

Moreover, medical education is starting to place greater emphasis on nutrition, equipping future healthcare providers with the knowledge and tools to guide patients toward healthier eating habits. Historically, medical schools have offered little training in nutrition, leaving doctors ill-prepared to address diet-related health issues. However, as the understanding of the link between food and health grows, more institutions are integrating nutrition education into their curricula.

In the future, we can expect to see a greater focus on personalized nutrition, where dietary recommendations are tailored to an individual's genetic makeup, microbiome, and unique health profile. Advances in technology, such as wearable devices and artificial intelligence, are also likely to play a role in helping people monitor their diet and make more informed choices based on real-time data about their health.

CONCLUSION: A PATH TOWARD HEALTHIER EATING

The concept of food as medicine is not a new one, but it is more relevant now than ever as the United States faces a health crisis fueled by poor dietary choices. By shifting the national conversation from treating diseases with medications to preventing them with food, we can begin to address the root causes of chronic illness and improve the health and well-being of millions of Americans.

DR. CRANDALL'S AMERICA:
The Power and Challenges of Food as Medicine

Throughout my career, I have seen the profound impact that food can have on health—both as a source of healing and, unfortunately, as a major contributor to disease. Time and time again, I've treated patients whose conditions were directly tied to their diets. What has struck me most is not just the preventable nature of many of these illnesses but also how deeply entrenched the barriers to better nutrition are for so many Americans.

One of my patients, a middle-aged woman named Susan, came to me with severe obesity, type 2 diabetes, and high blood pressure. She had been living on a diet of fast food and processed snacks for years, not because she didn't care about her health, but because she didn't have the knowledge or resources to make better choices. Susan lived in a food desert—an area where fresh fruits, vegetables, and whole foods were scarce. The nearest grocery store was miles away, and she didn't have reliable transportation. When I explained how changes in her diet could help her lose weight, lower her blood sugar, and reduce her risk of heart disease, she looked at me with a mixture of hope and despair. "Doctor, I don't even know where to start," she said.

Susan's story is not unique. I've met countless patients who know they need to eat healthier but are trapped in circumstances that make it nearly impossible. From the single mother juggling two jobs who relies on cheap, calorie-dense foods to the elderly man on a fixed income who can't afford fresh produce, the challenges are immense. And while I've seen some incredible transformations when patients are given the tools and support they need, I've also seen far too many cases where the system has failed them.

One success story I often think about is David, a man in his sixties who came to me after a near-fatal heart attack. David's diet had been a steady stream of fried foods, sugary drinks, and processed snacks. After his heart attack, he was determined to change. With guidance, he embraced a plant-based diet, started preparing his meals at home, and even began growing his own vegetables in a small garden. The change was remarkable—his cholesterol levels dropped, his blood pressure stabilized, and he regained a sense of control over his health. David's story is a testament to the power of food as medicine, but it also underscores the importance of education and support in making these changes sustainable.

Yet, for every David, there are patients like Maria, a young mother who struggled to change her family's eating habits. Despite her best efforts, the demands of her life made it difficult to prioritize healthy cooking. Maria told me, "I want to feed my kids better, but it's so much easier and cheaper to pick up something quick." Her story is a stark reminder that the structural and economic barriers to healthy eating remain a significant obstacle for many families.

As a doctor, these experiences have taught me that addressing diet-related diseases requires more than individual willpower—it requires systemic change. We need policies that make healthy food affordable and accessible. We need education programs that teach people how to cook and prepare nutritious meals. And we need to hold food manufacturers accountable for the role they play in promoting unhealthy diets.

I've also seen how cultural factors shape dietary habits. In my work as a medical missionary and anthropologist, I've observed communities that thrive on traditional diets rich in whole foods and fresh ingredients. These experiences have shown me what's possible when nutrition is prioritized, and they've fueled my frustration at the state of America's food system.

Still, there are glimmers of hope. I've seen schools introduce healthier lunch programs, communities establish farmers' markets in underserved areas, and patients reclaim their health by changing their diets. These efforts, while not yet widespread enough, remind me that change is possible. But to make a real difference, we must confront the systemic issues that keep healthy eating out of reach for so many Americans.

Through these stories, I've come to see food as one of the most powerful tools in medicine—a tool that has the potential to prevent and even reverse disease. But for food to truly serve as medicine, we need to create a society where healthy eating is not a privilege but a norm. The patients I've treated, and the challenges they've faced, have shown me both the urgency of this mission and the incredible potential for transformation when we prioritize nutrition in our approach to health.

R̲X̲ Dr. Crandall's Prescription for Using Food as Medicine

✔ **Incorporate More Anti-Inflammatory Foods.** Prioritize foods rich in antioxidants, such as berries, leafy greens, turmeric, and omega-3 fatty acids, to reduce inflammation and support overall health.

✔ **Use Herbs and Spices for Health Benefits.** Incorporate natural healing ingredients like ginger, garlic, cinnamon, and cayenne pepper to enhance flavor while boosting immunity and digestion.

✔ **Adopt a "Food First" Approach to Nutrition.** Focus on getting essential vitamins and minerals through whole foods rather than relying solely on supplements for nutrition.

✔ **Reduce Consumption of Artificial Additives.** Avoid foods containing artificial colors, preservatives, and flavor enhancers that may contribute to long-term health issues.

✔ **Practice Mindful Eating.** Slow down during meals, chew thoroughly, and pay attention to hunger and fullness cues to improve digestion and prevent overeating.

✔ **Explore Traditional Healing Diets.** Learn from cultures that emphasize whole foods and plant-based nutrition, such as the Mediterranean, Okinawan, or Ayurvedic diets, to find sustainable health practices.

✔ **Hydrate with Nutrient-Rich Beverages.** Replace sugary drinks with herbal teas, infused water, or bone broth to support digestion, hydration, and immune health.

Resources

Chauncey Crandall, M.D.
The Simple Heart Cure and Diet Plan: 28 Days of Healthy Meals and Over 100 Delicious and Easy Recipes
Humanix Books
The Mediterranean Diet Guide (www.Amazon.com).

Harvard School of Public Health
Provides a scientific breakdown of the diet and its benefits (https://nutritionsource.hsph.harvard.edu/healthy-weight/diet-reviews/mediterranean-diet/).

Blue Zones
Free recipes from the Blue Zones kitchen (https://www.bluezones.com/recipes/).

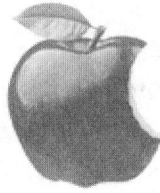

CHAPTER THREE

RETHINKING EXERCISE: MOVEMENT FOR EVERY BODY

P hysical activity has long been recognized as a cornerstone of good health, yet modern lifestyles and societal changes have made regular exercise a challenge for many Americans. Sedentary behavior has become the norm, driven by desk jobs, urban environments designed for cars rather than people, and the ever-present allure of digital entertainment. The result is an epidemic of physical inactivity, contributing to rising rates of obesity, heart disease, diabetes, and mental health issues. However, the path to better health doesn't require extreme workouts or expensive gym memberships. By rethinking exercise and embracing the idea that movement is for everybody, we can create a more inclusive, accessible, and sustainable approach to physical fitness.

THE IMPORTANCE OF PHYSICAL ACTIVITY FOR HEALTH AND LONGEVITY

Exercise is one of the most powerful tools for maintaining health, preventing disease, and promoting longevity. Regular physical activity supports cardiovascular health, strengthens muscles and bones, boosts mental well-being, and helps regulate weight. According to the Centers for Disease Control and Prevention (CDC), adults should aim for at least 150 minutes of moderate-intensity aerobic activity or 75 minutes of vigorous-intensity activity per week, along with muscle-strengthening exercises on two or more days. However, fewer than one in four adults in the United States meet these guidelines, and the consequences are far-reaching.

Physical inactivity is a major risk factor for a host of chronic diseases. Lack of exercise contributes to weight gain, which in turn increases the risk of heart disease, type 2 diabetes, and certain cancers. Regular physical activity, on the other hand, can reduce the risk of these conditions by improving blood pressure, lowering cholesterol levels, enhancing insulin sensitivity, and supporting healthy weight management. In addition to its physical benefits, exercise is a powerful tool for mental health. It reduces symptoms of anxiety and depression, improves mood, and enhances cognitive function.

Importantly, the benefits of exercise extend across all age groups and demographics. For children, physical activity supports healthy growth and development, while in older adults, it helps maintain mobility, balance, and independence. Despite the clear advantages, many people struggle to incorporate regular movement into their lives, often due to misconceptions about what exercise should look like.

DEBUNKING COMMON EXERCISE MYTHS

One of the biggest barriers to physical activity is the misconception that exercise must be intense or time-consuming or require a gym membership. These myths can discourage people from getting started, especially if they feel that they don't have the time, resources, or physical ability to participate in traditional fitness routines.

Myth #1: You need a gym to get fit.

While gyms offer a variety of equipment and classes, they are by no means essential for achieving fitness. Many people believe that a gym membership is a prerequisite for getting in shape, but this couldn't be further from the truth. Bodyweight exercises, walking, running, cycling, swimming, and yoga are all effective ways to stay fit without ever setting foot in a gym. These forms of exercise can be done at home, in local parks, or even at work during breaks. The key is finding activities that are enjoyable and sustainable over the long term.

Myth #2: You have to work out for long periods to see results.

Another common misconception is that exercise must last for an hour or more to be beneficial. In reality, short bursts of physical activity can be just as effective, especially for those with busy schedules. Research has shown that even 10- to 15-minute sessions of moderate to vigorous exercise, repeated throughout the day, can improve cardiovascular health, boost metabolism, and promote weight loss. High-intensity interval training (HIIT), for example, is a time-efficient way to burn calories and build strength in just 20 to 30 minutes.

Myth #3: Exercise has to be intense to be effective.

Many people associate exercise with sweat-drenched, heart-pounding workouts, but moderate-intensity activities can offer significant health benefits as well. Walking, dancing, gardening, and cycling at a leisurely pace are all forms of physical activity that elevate the heart rate and promote cardiovascular health. The key is consistency—moving your body regularly is more important than the intensity of any single workout. For people who are new to exercise or have physical limitations, low-impact activities such as swimming, yoga, or tai chi can be a great starting point.

ACCESSIBLE WAYS TO INCORPORATE MOVEMENT INTO DAILY LIFE

For many Americans, especially those with demanding jobs or family responsibilities, finding time for formal exercise can be challenging. However, by shifting the focus from structured workouts to movement in general, it becomes easier to incorporate physical activity into daily routines. Everyday tasks, when approached mindfully, can offer opportunities for movement.

Walking is one of the simplest and most accessible forms of exercise. Whether it's taking the stairs instead of the elevator, walking or biking to work, or going for a walk during lunch breaks, these small changes can add up. Aiming for 10,000 steps per day—a goal popularized by fitness trackers—is a good benchmark for promoting overall health and increasing daily activity levels.

Stretching and *mobility exercises* are often overlooked but are essential for maintaining flexibility, reducing the risk of injury, and improving posture. Incorporating simple stretches into the day, such as standing up to stretch after long periods of sitting or doing gentle yoga poses before bed, can make a big difference.

Functional fitness refers to exercises that mimic everyday movements, helping to build strength and improve coordination in ways that support daily activities. Squatting, lifting, pushing, and pulling are all movements that we perform in daily life, and they can be enhanced through exercises that focus on these motions. Bodyweight exercises like squats, lunges, push-ups, and planks are excellent examples of functional fitness that can be done anywhere.

Incorporating *"exercise snacks"*—short bursts of activity throughout the day—is another effective way to stay active. These could include standing up to do a few squats, doing jumping jacks during TV commercials, or taking a brisk walk around the office during a break. This approach helps break up sedentary time and increases overall daily activity levels without the need for long workout sessions.

HOW CITIES AND WORKPLACES CAN PROMOTE ACTIVE LIVING

The environments in which we live and work play a critical role in shaping our activity levels. Urban planning, transportation infrastructure, and workplace culture all influence how much movement we engage in throughout the day. By designing cities and workplaces with physical activity in mind, we can create environments that make it easier for people to stay active.

Walkable cities are key to promoting daily movement. Cities that prioritize pedestrian-friendly streets, bike lanes, public parks, and green spaces encourage people to walk or bike instead of driving. In contrast, car-dependent cities with few sidewalks or bike paths make it difficult for residents to engage in active transportation. Urban planners can help reverse the trend of sedentary living by designing neighborhoods that make walking and biking safe, convenient, and enjoyable.

Workplaces also have a role to play in supporting employee health and well-being. Many office jobs involve long hours of sitting, which has been linked to numerous health problems, including obesity, heart disease, and even early death. Companies can encourage movement by offering standing desks, holding walking meetings, or creating spaces for employees to stretch or exercise during breaks. Some companies have also implemented wellness programs that offer fitness classes, gym memberships, or incentives for employees who meet activity goals.

Public policies can further support active living by investing in public transportation, parks, and recreation programs. Governments can also implement initiatives such as "open streets" events, where city streets are closed to cars for a day, allowing residents to walk, bike, or play. In addition, schools and community organizations can promote physical activity through sports leagues, after-school programs, and outdoor recreation activities.

PROFILES OF PROGRAMS SUCCESSFULLY GETTING PEOPLE MOVING

There are numerous examples of programs and initiatives that have successfully encouraged physical activity in diverse populations. These programs often focus on making exercise fun, accessible, and integrated into daily life.

One such program is parkrun, a global initiative that organizes free, weekly, timed 5K runs in local parks. Parkrun events are open to people of all ages and fitness levels, and they are designed to be non-competitive, emphasizing participation and community rather than performance. The accessibility of parkrun—participants can walk, jog, or run—has made it a popular way for people to stay active, especially in communities where traditional fitness opportunities may be limited.

Blue Zones projects, inspired by areas of the world where people live the longest, have focused on redesigning communities to encourage movement. In cities like Albert Lea, Minnesota, and Fort Worth, Texas, Blue Zones initiatives have improved walkability, increased access to parks and recreational facilities, and implemented school and workplace wellness programs. These changes have resulted in measurable improvements in physical activity levels, as well as reductions in obesity and chronic disease rates.

Incorporating exercise into schools is another way to promote lifelong physical activity. The SPARK (Sports, Play, and Active

Recreation for Kids) program, for example, has been implemented in schools across the United States to increase the quantity and quality of physical education. By focusing on fun, inclusive, and active PE classes, SPARK has improved fitness levels among students and helped establish healthy habits early in life.

For older adults, programs like SilverSneakers offer free or low-cost fitness classes tailored to seniors. These classes focus on improving strength, balance, and flexibility, helping older adults stay active and independent. SilverSneakers classes are offered in community centers and gyms, and even online, making them accessible to a wide range of participants.

CONCLUSION: MOVEMENT FOR EVERY BODY

The message is clear: movement is for everybody. It doesn't matter if you're young or old, fit or unfit—physical activity is essential for maintaining health, preventing disease, and improving quality of life.

DR. CRANDALL'S AMERICA:
The Challenge of Rethinking Exercise

As a cardiologist and preventive medicine physician, I've seen how transformative physical activity can be for my patients. But I've also witnessed the obstacles that keep so many Americans from embracing movement in their daily lives. Throughout my career, I've dealt with patients who struggle with the idea of exercise—not because they don't understand its importance, but because their lives are filled with barriers that make regular physical activity seem out of reach.

One of my patients, James, was a 48-year-old father of three who came to me with severe hypertension and early signs of heart disease. When I asked about his exercise routine, he shook his head and said, "Doctor, I don't have time for that. Between work and my kids, I'm lucky if I get five minutes to myself." James's story is all too common. Many patients feel overwhelmed by the demands of daily life, leaving little room for self-care. For James, the idea of exercise felt like an additional burden, not a solution.

We started small. I suggested that he take a 10-minute walk during his lunch break and spend 15 minutes playing outside with his kids in the evenings. Over time, those small steps grew into a habit. He began walking daily, eventually incorporating light jogging and even family bike rides. A year later, James returned for a follow-up, and the transformation was striking. His blood pressure was under control, he'd lost weight, and, most importantly, he told me, "I feel like I've got more energy to be there for my family." Stories like James's remind me of the power of starting small and making exercise feel achievable.

But not all patients have the same outcome. I think of Maria, a 62-year-old woman with obesity and diabetes who was struggling with severe joint pain. "Doctor, I can barely get out of bed some days," she told me. For Maria, traditional exercise routines felt impossible, and her condition only worsened as her mobility declined. We worked together to find gentle, low-impact activities like chair exercises and water aerobics, but her progress was slow. Maria's case highlights a harsh truth: for many Americans, health challenges compound over time, making it harder to break the cycle and adopt healthier habits.

I've also seen how socioeconomic factors limit access to physical activity. In low-income neighborhoods, where I've worked as both a physician and a medical missionary, the lack of safe spaces to exercise is a persistent issue.

One patient, a young mother named Alisha, lived in an area with no sidewalks or parks. She told me, "I'd love to take my kids outside more, but it's just not safe." Her story underscores the critical role that community design and infrastructure play in promoting or hindering physical activity.

On the other hand, I've been inspired by communities that come together to create opportunities for movement. In one rural town where I volunteered, a group of church members started a weekly walking club that grew into a full-fledged health initiative, complete with fitness classes and community events. Seeing the joy and camaraderie that emerged from these gatherings was a powerful reminder of how movement can bring people together and improve health in the process.

Despite the challenges, I remain optimistic. I've seen firsthand how even small changes can lead to significant improvements in health and quality of life. But the barriers my patients face are a stark reminder that promoting exercise requires more than just individual effort—it requires systemic change. We need safe parks, walkable neighborhoods, and affordable fitness programs. We need workplaces and schools that encourage movement throughout the day. And we need to shift the narrative around exercise from being a chore to being a natural and enjoyable part of life.

Through these stories, I've learned that rethinking exercise means meeting people where they are and helping them find ways to move that fit into their lives. It's not about perfection; it's about progress. And when patients like James or communities like that rural town embrace the idea of movement for everybody, it reaffirms my belief that we can create a healthier, more active America.

R℞ Dr. Crandall's Prescription for Rethinking Exercise

✔ **Incorporate Movement Throughout the Day.** Instead of limiting exercise to structured workouts, integrate movement into daily life through activities like stretching, standing breaks, and short walks.

✔ **Experiment with Different Types of Exercise.** Find physical activities that suit your body and interests, such as dance, swimming, martial arts, or resistance training, to stay engaged and motivated.

✔ **Prioritize Mobility and Flexibility Training.** Include stretching, yoga, or dynamic warm-ups to maintain joint health, reduce injury risk, and improve overall movement efficiency.

✔ **Turn Daily Chores into Exercise Opportunities.** Tasks like gardening, carrying groceries, or house cleaning can serve as functional fitness activities that contribute to an active lifestyle.

✔ **Adopt an "Every Bit Counts" Mindset.** Understand that small movements, such as taking the stairs instead of the elevator or parking farther away, add up and contribute to long-term health benefits.

✔ **Set Performance-Based Rather Than Just Weight-Loss Goals.** Focus on goals like increasing endurance, lifting heavier weights, or improving flexibility rather than relying solely on the scale for motivation.

✔ **Make Exercise a Social Activity.** Join a fitness class, walking group, or recreational sports league to stay accountable, build community, and make movement more enjoyable.

Resources

Physical Activity Guidelines for Americans
Science-based recommendations to help individuals improve their health through regular physical activity (https://odphp.health.gov/our-work/nutrition-physical-activity/physical-activity-guidelines).

Silver Sneakers
A fitness program for seniors that is generally accessed through Medicare and Medicare Advantage Plans (https://tools.silversneakers.com).

Move Your Way Campaign (HHS)
Free workout videos and tips (https://odphp.health.gov/our-work/nutrition-physical-activity/move-your-way-community-resources).

YMCA
Many YMCA locations offer gym access, group fitness classes, swimming, and family activities (www.ymca.org).

Parks and Recreation Programs
Most municipalities offer free or affordable fitness programs in local parks or other recreational sites. Contact your local municipality.

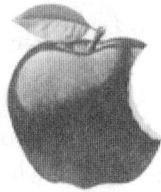

CHAPTER FOUR

MENTAL HEALTH
MATTERS

In recent years, mental health has emerged as one of the most pressing public health issues in the United States and globally. Mental health disorders, including anxiety, depression, and stress-related conditions, affect millions of people across all demographics and are a leading cause of disability, decreased quality of life, and even mortality. Despite growing awareness of the mental health crisis, the stigma surrounding mental illness persists, and access to care remains a challenge for many. Addressing the mental health epidemic is not only a matter of providing more services but also changing how society views mental health and prioritizes emotional well-being.

The mental health crisis in America has many contributing factors, from the fast pace of modern life and increasing economic pressures to the rise of social media and the ongoing impact of the COVID-19 pandemic. This chapter explores the mental health challenges facing the country, the factors that contribute to poor mental well-being, and the holistic approaches that can help individuals and communities improve their mental health.

THE MENTAL HEALTH EPIDEMIC IN AMERICA

Mental health disorders are alarmingly common in the United States. According to the National Institute of Mental Health (NIMH), nearly one in five U.S. adults—about 51.5 million people—experienced mental illness in 2020. These conditions ranged from mild to severe and included anxiety disorders, depression, post-traumatic stress disorder (PTSD), bipolar disorder, and schizophrenia, among others. While many people experience mild symptoms that may not interfere significantly with daily life, a significant portion of the population—roughly 13 million adults—live with serious mental illness, which severely impairs their ability to function.

In addition to these numbers, mental health problems are on the rise, particularly among young people. The U.S. Surgeon General has declared youth mental health a national crisis, noting that the number of adolescents experiencing feelings of persistent sadness or hopelessness has increased by 40% in the past decade. Suicide is now the second leading cause of death among individuals aged 10 to 34, highlighting the urgent need for better mental health support systems for young people.

The COVID-19 pandemic has only exacerbated the situation. The isolation, uncertainty, and stress caused by the pandemic led to a sharp increase in mental health issues. Surveys conducted during the pandemic showed that nearly half of U.S. adults reported struggling with anxiety or depression. For many, the loss of loved ones, economic hardships, and the disruption of daily life created a perfect storm for mental health challenges. While the pandemic amplified pre-existing problems, it also revealed the systemic weaknesses in the country's mental health care system.

IMPACT OF MODERN LIFESTYLES ON MENTAL HEALTH

Several elements of modern life contribute to the mental health crisis. Stress, social isolation, and the pressures of balancing work, family, and personal well-being are taking a toll on people's mental health. As society becomes more fast-paced, digitally connected, and economically competitive, the toll on mental well-being has grown significantly.

One of the primary drivers of mental health challenges is *chronic stress*. The constant demands of work, financial pressures, and the expectations to be constantly available and productive have left many Americans feeling overwhelmed. The rise of the gig economy and the blurring lines between work and personal time have contributed to a culture of overwork and burnout. Chronic stress can lead to anxiety, depression, sleep problems, and a weakened immune system, and it can also exacerbate existing mental health conditions.

Social isolation is another major factor affecting mental well-being. While technology has made it easier than ever to connect with others, it has also replaced many face-to-face interactions with virtual ones. Studies have shown that despite the increase in digital communication, people are feeling lonelier than ever. This paradox of hyperconnectivity and isolation has profound implications for mental health, as human beings are social creatures who thrive on meaningful, in-person interactions.

Social media has a significant impact on mental health, especially among adolescents and young adults. While platforms like Instagram, TikTok, and Twitter allow users to connect with friends and access information, they can also foster feelings of inadequacy, anxiety, and depression. The constant comparison to curated, idealized versions of others' lives can create a sense of pressure to meet unrealistic standards of beauty, success, and happiness. Additionally, the addictive nature of social media, with its endless scrolling and notifications, can disrupt sleep, contribute to anxiety, and exacerbate mental health issues.

Economic inequality and *financial insecurity* are also key factors in the mental health crisis. Research has shown that individuals in lower socioeconomic brackets are more likely to experience stress, anxiety, and depression. Economic hardships, including unemployment, housing instability, and food insecurity, create chronic stress that can erode mental well-being over time. In the United States, where access to mental health services is often linked to employment and insurance coverage, those who are most in need of support are often the least likely to receive it.

THE STIGMA AROUND MENTAL HEALTH

Despite the prevalence of mental health issues, stigma continues to be a major barrier to seeking help. Many people still view mental illness as a sign of weakness or something to be ashamed of, which prevents them from reaching out for the support they need. This stigma is often perpetuated by cultural norms, misconceptions about mental illness, and a lack of education around the topic.

For example, men are often socialized to believe that they must be strong, stoic, and self-reliant, which can make it difficult for them to admit when they are struggling. As a result, men are less likely to seek mental health treatment, even though they are just as likely as women to experience mental health issues. This reluctance to seek help can lead to untreated mental health problems, higher rates of substance abuse, and, tragically, higher suicide rates among men.

In addition, certain cultural and ethnic groups may face unique stigmas around mental health. For example, in some Asian, Latino, and African American communities, mental health issues may be seen as something that should be kept private, or they may be misunderstood as spiritual or moral failings rather than medical conditions. This cultural stigma can create additional barriers to seeking treatment, even when mental health services are available.

Combatting stigma requires a multi-faceted approach. Education is key to breaking down misconceptions about mental illness and normalizing the conversation around mental health. Public awareness campaigns, such as those launched by organizations like the National Alliance on Mental Illness (NAMI) and Mental Health America (MHA), can help reduce stigma by sharing personal stories, providing information about mental health conditions, and encouraging individuals to seek help.

HOLISTIC APPROACHES TO MENTAL HEALTH

Addressing mental health requires a holistic approach that considers not just the mind, but the body and the environment as well. While traditional treatments like therapy and medication are essential tools in managing mental health conditions, they are most effective when combined with lifestyle changes that promote overall well-being.

Therapy remains one of the most effective treatments for mental health disorders. Cognitive-behavioral therapy (CBT), for example, has been shown to be particularly effective for conditions like anxiety and depression. CBT helps individuals identify and challenge negative thought patterns and develop healthier ways of thinking and coping. Other forms of therapy, such as psychotherapy, dialectical behavior therapy (DBT), and trauma-focused therapies, can also be effective, depending on the individual's needs.

However, therapy is often out of reach for many people due to cost, lack of insurance coverage, or a shortage of mental health professionals in their area. Teletherapy, which became more widespread during the COVID-19 pandemic, has expanded access to mental health care by allowing individuals to receive therapy remotely. This is especially beneficial for those living in rural areas or who may not feel comfortable seeking in-person therapy.

Mindfulness and meditation are increasingly recognized as powerful tools for managing stress and improving mental health. These practices encourage individuals to focus on the present moment, become more aware of their thoughts and feelings, and develop a sense of calm and clarity. Research has shown that mindfulness-based interventions can reduce symptoms of anxiety, depression, and PTSD, as well as improve overall emotional regulation.

Exercise is another critical component of mental health. Regular physical activity has been shown to reduce symptoms of depression and anxiety, improve mood, and increase feelings of well-being. Exercise releases endorphins—chemicals in the brain that act as natural mood elevators—and can also provide a sense of accomplishment and improved self-esteem. Importantly, even moderate amounts of exercise, such as walking or yoga, can have a positive impact on mental health.

Social connections are vital for mental well-being. Strong relationships with family, friends, and community members provide emotional support, reduce feelings of loneliness, and help individuals cope with stress. Engaging in social activities, joining support groups, or participating in community events can help foster a sense of belonging and reduce the isolation that often accompanies mental health challenges.

Nutrition also plays a significant role in mental health. A growing body of research suggests that diet can influence mood and mental health, with poor nutrition being linked to a higher risk of mental health disorders. Diets high in processed foods, sugar, and unhealthy fats can contribute to inflammation in the body, which is associated with depression and anxiety. On the other hand, diets rich in fruits, vegetables, whole grains, lean proteins, and omega-3 fatty acids have been shown to support brain health and reduce the risk of mental health conditions.

POLICY RECOMMENDATIONS FOR IMPROVING MENTAL HEALTH SERVICES

Addressing the mental health crisis in the United States will require systemic changes to improve access to care, reduce stigma, and integrate mental health services into primary care settings. Several policy recommendations can help create a more robust mental health system.

Expanding access to mental health services is crucial. This can be done by increasing funding for mental health programs, expanding insurance coverage for mental health care, and addressing the shortage of mental health professionals in underserved areas. Teletherapy should be made a permanent option for those who prefer or need it.

DR. CRANDALL'S AMERICA:
The Growing Mental Health Crisis

Throughout my career, I've seen the deep connection between physical and mental health—and how often the latter is overlooked in our healthcare system. The stories of my patients have shown me that while mental health challenges have always existed, the pressures of modern life are making these issues more widespread and severe. At the same time, I've also seen the incredible resilience of the human spirit when people are given the tools and support they need to heal.

One of my patients, Michael, was a 42-year-old executive who came to me complaining of chest pain and difficulty breathing. After running a series of tests, I was relieved to find that his heart was in good condition. But when I asked about his stress levels, he broke down in tears. "I feel like I'm drowning," he admitted. Michael was experiencing a classic anxiety disorder, brought on by the relentless demands of his job and personal life. His story is one I've encountered countless times—physical symptoms that are the manifestation of untreated mental health issues. For Michael, the solution wasn't a pill or procedure;

it was learning to manage his stress through therapy, mindfulness practices, and setting healthier boundaries in his life. Over time, he regained control, and his physical symptoms disappeared.

Unfortunately, not all cases are as clear-cut. I once treated a teenager named Emily who was struggling with depression. She had been diagnosed with obesity and prediabetes, conditions that had eroded her self-esteem and left her feeling isolated. "It's like I'm stuck in this cycle," she told me. "I don't feel good about myself, so I eat more, and then I feel worse." Emily's story broke my heart because it highlighted how intertwined mental and physical health can be. We worked together to address both her physical and emotional well-being, but progress was slow. Her case reminded me of how urgently we need to integrate mental health care into every aspect of medicine.

The stigma surrounding mental health continues to be one of the biggest barriers I see. One of my older patients, a retired factory worker named Bill, struggled with severe depression after the death of his wife. When I suggested therapy, he brushed it off. "I'm not crazy, Doc. I just need to tough it out," he said. His resistance was a stark reminder of the cultural attitudes that prevent many people, especially older generations, from seeking the help they need. Eventually, with gentle encouragement and the involvement of his family, Bill agreed to see a counselor, and his quality of life improved dramatically.

Yet, there are moments of hope. I've seen schools implement programs to teach children mindfulness and stress management skills. I've watched workplaces adopt wellness initiatives that prioritize employee mental health. And I've worked with community organizations that provide free or low-cost therapy to those in need. These efforts, while still limited, show that progress is possible.

However, the systemic challenges remain daunting. Many of my patients have struggled to access mental health care due to cost, long wait times, or a lack of providers in their area. One young mother, Sarah, told me she had to wait three months for her first therapy appointment. "By the time I got in, I didn't even know what to say anymore," she said. Stories like hers illustrate why we need urgent reforms to make mental health care more accessible and integrated into primary care.

As a doctor, I've learned that addressing mental health isn't just about treating symptoms—it's about creating a culture that values emotional well-being as much as physical health. It's about asking the right questions, listening without judgment, and providing patients with the resources they need to heal. And it's about advocating for systemic changes that ensure that everyone, regardless of their background or circumstances, has access to the care they deserve.

Through these stories, I've come to understand that while the mental health crisis is growing, so too is our ability to address it. With compassion, innovation, and a commitment to breaking down barriers, we can help our patients find their way back to a healthier, more balanced life. It won't happen overnight, but every success—every Michael, Emily, or Bill—reminds me that progress is not only possible but essential.

℞ Dr. Crandall's Prescription for Better Mental Health

- **Establish a Daily Mental Wellness Routine.** Incorporate activities like meditation, journaling, or deep breathing exercises to support emotional resilience and stress management.
- **Develop Healthy Sleep Habits.** Prioritize a consistent sleep schedule, reduce screen time before bed, and create a calming bedtime routine to support mental clarity and emotional stability.
- **Recognize the Connection Between Diet and Mental Health.** Consume nutrient-dense foods rich in omega-3s, magnesium, and B vitamins to support brain function and mood regulation.
- **Set Healthy Boundaries in Relationships.** Learn to say no, limit exposure to toxic individuals, and prioritize interactions that contribute positively to mental well-being.
- **Engage in Purposeful Activities.** Pursue hobbies, volunteer work, or creative outlets that provide a sense of fulfillment and reduce stress levels.
- **Practice Digital Detoxing.** Take breaks from social media and excessive news consumption to prevent anxiety, information overload, and negative comparisons.
- **Seek Professional Support Without Stigma.** Understand that therapy, counseling, or support groups are valuable resources that can provide guidance, coping strategies, and emotional support.

Resources

National Alliance on Mental Illness (NAMI)
Education, advocacy, support groups, and a free helpline (1-800-950-NAMI [6264]; https://www.nami.org).

Substance Abuse and Mental Health Services Administration (SAMHSA)
Programs and treatment locators, along with crisis and suicide hotlines (1-800-662-HELP [4357]; https://www.samhsa.gov).

Centers for Disease Control and Prevention Mental Health Resources (CDC)
Information on public health initiatives, stress, community resources, mental health stigma, and more (https://www.cdc.gov/mental-health/index.html).

American Foundation for Suicide Prevention (AFSP)
Research, prevention, and support, along with resources for people who have lost loved ones to suicide (https://afsp.org).

National Institute on Aging (NIA)
Offers a comprehensive Social Isolation and Loneliness Outreach Toolkit, with free publications, graphics, and resources aimed at increasing connectedness among older adults (https://www.nia.nih.gov/toolkits/social-isolation).

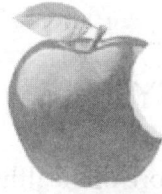

CHAPTER FIVE

A NEW HEALTHCARE PARADIGM

The American healthcare system is at a critical juncture. Despite being one of the most advanced healthcare systems in the world, it faces serious challenges, including soaring costs, uneven access, and an overemphasis on treating disease rather than preventing it. The current system often prioritizes reactive treatments over proactive, preventive care, resulting in an unsustainable cycle of escalating medical expenses and worsening health outcomes. As chronic diseases like heart disease, diabetes, and cancer continue to rise, the need for a new healthcare paradigm has never been more urgent.

This chapter explores the limitations of the existing U.S. healthcare system, the benefits of shifting toward a prevention-focused model, and examples of successful healthcare systems around the world. It will also discuss how healthcare policy can be reshaped to prioritize long-term health outcomes, increase access to care, and reduce the overall burden of disease.

THE CHALLENGES OF THE
U.S. HEALTHCARE SYSTEM

The United States spends more on healthcare than any other nation, yet it lags behind other high-income countries in key health outcomes such as life expectancy, infant mortality, and the prevalence of chronic disease. According to data from the Centers for Medicare & Medicaid Services (CMS), the U.S. healthcare system accounted for nearly 18% of the country's GDP in 2021, amounting to over $4 trillion in annual expenditures. Despite this massive investment, millions of Americans are uninsured or underinsured, and many more struggle to afford necessary medical care.

One of the primary reasons for this disconnect between spending and outcomes is the *focus on treatment rather than prevention*. The current healthcare system is largely reactive, meaning that it focuses on diagnosing and treating illnesses after they occur rather than taking steps to prevent them in the first place. This approach is particularly evident in the management of chronic diseases, which account for 90% of the nation's healthcare costs. Conditions like heart disease, diabetes, and cancer are often treated with medications and surgeries rather than lifestyle changes that could prevent or even reverse the progression of disease.

Another major challenge is *uneven access to care*. The U.S. healthcare system is highly fragmented, with significant disparities in access to healthcare services based on factors like income, geography, and race. Rural communities often lack access to healthcare providers, forcing residents to travel long distances to receive care. Low-income individuals and people of color are more likely to be uninsured or underinsured, which limits their ability to seek timely medical care. Even those with insurance may face high deductibles, co-pays, and out-of-pocket expenses that make it difficult to afford necessary treatments.

Additionally, the healthcare system often prioritizes *acute care over long-term health management*. Emergency rooms, for example, are frequently used as primary care facilities by individuals who do not have access to regular healthcare services. This not only leads to higher healthcare costs but also results in suboptimal care for managing chronic conditions. Instead of focusing on preventive care and early interventions, the system tends to focus on managing acute health crises after they occur, which often leads to worse outcomes and higher costs.

THE NEED FOR A PREVENTIVE APPROACH TO HEALTHCARE

To address the limitations of the current system, a shift toward preventive care is essential. Preventive healthcare emphasizes early detection, health education, and lifestyle interventions to reduce the risk of developing chronic diseases. This approach not only improves health outcomes but also reduces healthcare costs by minimizing the need for expensive treatments down the line.

One of the key advantages of preventive care is its *cost-effectiveness*. For example, studies have shown that investing in preventive measures such as smoking cessation programs, vaccination campaigns, and regular health screenings can save millions of dollars in medical expenses. Early detection of diseases like cancer or diabetes allows for less invasive and less costly treatments, while lifestyle interventions like promoting physical activity and healthy eating can prevent the onset of these diseases altogether.

Preventive care also focuses on the *social determinants of health*— the conditions in which people live, work, and age that impact their health outcomes. Addressing social determinants like access to healthy food, safe housing, clean air, and education can significantly improve public health. For instance, ensuring that communities have access to affordable, fresh produce can help reduce rates of obesity and diabetes, while improving air quality can lower the incidence of respiratory diseases like asthma.

Moreover, a prevention-focused healthcare system places greater emphasis on *patient education and empowerment*. By teaching individuals how to manage their health through diet, exercise, and other lifestyle changes, healthcare providers can help reduce the reliance on medications and surgeries. Patients who are actively involved in their health decisions are more likely to make positive choices and adhere to recommended treatments, leading to better long-term outcomes.

SUCCESSFUL HEALTHCARE MODELS THAT PRIORITIZE PREVENTION

Several countries around the world have adopted healthcare models that emphasize prevention and long-term health outcomes, and the results are impressive. These systems offer valuable lessons for the United States as it seeks to reform its healthcare approach.

One of the most notable examples is the National Health Service (NHS) in the United Kingdom. The NHS provides universal healthcare coverage, ensuring that all residents have access to medical care regardless of income. The NHS places a strong emphasis on primary care, with general practitioners (GPs) serving as the first point of contact for most patients. GPs play a crucial role in preventive care by conducting regular check-ups, offering vaccinations, and providing health education. Additionally, the NHS invests in public health campaigns that promote healthy behaviors, such as reducing alcohol consumption and encouraging physical activity.

In Denmark, the healthcare system is also centered on prevention and primary care. Danish citizens have access to free healthcare services, including preventive screenings, vaccinations, and lifestyle counseling. The government invests heavily in public health programs, such as initiatives to reduce smoking rates and promote cycling as a means of transportation. Denmark's focus on preventive care has led to lower rates of chronic diseases like heart disease and diabetes, compared to many other countries.

Singapore offers another example of a healthcare system that balances affordability with quality care. The government of Singapore provides universal healthcare coverage while promoting personal responsibility for health. Singapore's healthcare model is known for its emphasis on cost control and efficiency, with a strong focus on preventive care. The government encourages healthy lifestyles through public health campaigns, subsidies for gym memberships, and incentives for individuals to undergo regular health screenings. As a result, Singapore has some of the lowest rates of chronic disease and one of the highest life expectancies in the world.

In Cuba, prevention is a fundamental pillar of the healthcare system. Cuban healthcare is characterized by its community-based approach, where doctors are assigned to specific neighborhoods and are responsible for the health of the residents in their assigned areas. These doctors focus on early detection, preventive care, and patient education. Cuba's emphasis on preventive healthcare has led to impressive health outcomes, including lower infant mortality rates and higher life expectancy, compared to many wealthier nations.

HOW HEALTHCARE POLICY CAN BE RESHAPED TO PRIORITIZE LONG-TERM HEALTH OUTCOMES

For the United States to adopt a more preventive approach to healthcare, significant changes are needed in both policy and practice. Several key reforms can help reshape the healthcare system to focus on long-term health outcomes rather than short-term fixes.

Expand Access to Primary Care

Primary care providers play a critical role in preventive healthcare. By expanding access to primary care services, more individuals can receive regular check-ups, screenings, and health education. One way to achieve this is by increasing funding for community health centers, which provide affordable primary care services to underserved populations. Additionally, incentivizing medical students to pursue careers in primary care—especially in rural and low-income areas—can help address the shortage of primary care providers.

Integrate Preventive Care into Health Insurance Plans

Health insurance plans should prioritize preventive services, such as vaccinations, screenings, and lifestyle counseling. Under the Affordable Care Act (ACA), many preventive services are already covered without cost-sharing for patients, but more can be done to expand coverage. For example, insurance plans could provide additional incentives for individuals who engage in healthy behaviors, such as participating in smoking cessation programs or undergoing regular health screenings. Expanding access to mental health services, which are often excluded from preventive care discussions, is also crucial.

Address Social Determinants of Health

Healthcare policy must take into account the social determinants of health that contribute to poor outcomes. Policies that improve access to nutritious food, affordable housing, clean air, and safe environments are essential for promoting public health. For example, expanding funding for programs like the Supplemental Nutrition Assistance Program (SNAP) and the Women, Infants, and Children (WIC) program can help reduce food insecurity, while investments in affordable housing can reduce the stress and health problems associated with housing instability.

Invest in Public Health Campaigns

Public health campaigns that promote healthy behaviors can play a significant role in preventing chronic diseases. Government agencies, schools, and community organizations should collaborate on initiatives that encourage physical activity, healthy eating, and mental well-being. For example, campaigns that promote walking or biking to work, reducing sugar intake, or quitting smoking can help shift public attitudes and behaviors toward healthier choices.

Shift Reimbursement Models to Value-Based Care

One of the most significant challenges in the current U.S. healthcare system is the fee-for-service model, which incentivizes providers to perform more tests and procedures rather than focusing on patient outcomes. Shifting to a value-based care model, where providers are reimbursed based on the quality of care and patient outcomes, would encourage healthcare providers to focus more on prevention and long-term health management. In a value-based care system, healthcare providers are rewarded for keeping patients healthy, rather than for the volume of services they provide.

CONCLUSION: A PATH TOWARD A HEALTHIER FUTURE

The current U.S. healthcare system, with its focus on reactive treatment and acute care, is unsustainable. Rising costs, increasing rates of chronic disease, and uneven access to care have created an urgent need for change. A new healthcare paradigm, one that prioritizes preventive care and long-term health outcomes, offers a promising path forward.

By expanding access to primary care, integrating preventive services into health insurance, addressing social determinants of health, and investing in public health initiatives, the United States can create a healthcare system that promotes well-being and reduces the burden of disease. Successful models from other countries demonstrate that prioritizing prevention leads to better health outcomes, lower costs, and a healthier population.

The time has come for the United States to shift its focus from treating diseases to preventing them, creating a healthcare system that serves everyone's long-term health needs.

DR. CRANDALL'S AMERICA:
The Need for a New Healthcare Paradigm

As a doctor, I've spent years navigating a healthcare system that often feels reactive rather than preventive. Time and again, I've seen patients enter my office with conditions that could have been prevented had they received the right guidance, resources, or interventions earlier in their lives. The current system frequently prioritizes treating illness over promoting wellness, and the consequences are written in the stories of my patients.

One such patient was Richard, a 60-year-old man who came to me after suffering his second heart attack. He'd been living with hypertension, high cholesterol, and type 2 diabetes for years, all of which had been managed with medication but never addressed holistically. "I feel like I'm just taking pills and waiting for the next bad thing to happen," he admitted. Richard's case was a classic example of how our system focuses on managing symptoms rather than addressing root causes. When we worked together to overhaul his diet, incorporate regular exercise, and reduce his stress, he began to see real progress—not just in his numbers but in how he felt every day. "Why didn't someone tell me this earlier?" he asked. His frustration was valid, and I've heard similar sentiments from countless patients over the years.

Then there's the story of Gloria, a 45-year-old single mother who came to me with advanced kidney disease. She had struggled with untreated high blood pressure for years, a condition she didn't fully understand because she hadn't had consistent access to primary care. "I couldn't afford to go to the doctor unless it was an emergency," she told me. Gloria's situation highlights a painful truth: Our healthcare system often fails the people who need it most. Preventive care could have made all the difference for her, but instead, she was now facing a lifelong struggle with a chronic condition that would require dialysis and possibly a transplant.

Despite these challenges, I've also seen glimmers of hope—moments where a shift toward a more preventive model of care has made a tangible difference. I think of a community health clinic I volunteered at early in my career, where a team of doctors, dietitians, and social workers worked together to address not just physical health but the underlying factors contributing to illness. Patients there didn't just receive prescriptions; they received education, counseling, and support to make lasting changes. Watching patients thrive in that environment gave me a glimpse of what healthcare could be if we prioritize prevention.

One of the most inspiring examples I've witnessed came from a corporate wellness program that focused on empowering employees to take charge of their health. One participant, a man named Derek, was on the brink of developing diabetes. Through a combination of health coaching, access to nutritious meals at work, and regular exercise sessions, Derek reversed his prediabetes entirely. "I never thought I could feel this good," he told me. His story is proof that when we invest in prevention, the rewards are significant—not just for individuals but for communities and workplaces as a whole.

However, these bright spots are exceptions, not the rule. The majority of my patients come to me after years of unmanaged or poorly managed health issues. Our healthcare system often prioritizes acute care and crisis management, leaving little room for the proactive measures that could prevent those crises in the first place. Insurance reimbursement structures rarely incentivize doctors to spend time on patient education or preventive care, creating a system that perpetuates the cycle of reactive treatment.

I've also seen the strain this system places on providers. Many of my colleagues express frustration at the time constraints and administrative burdens that keep them from focusing on their patients' long-term well-being. Burnout among healthcare professionals is rising, and it's a reflection of a system that often feels at odds with the very mission of healing.

These stories underscore the need for a paradigm shift in healthcare—one that prioritizes prevention, addresses social determinants of health, and empowers patients to take an active role in their own wellness. Through my experiences, I've come to believe that this shift is not only necessary but achievable. It will require systemic changes, from how we train doctors to how we reimburse care, but the potential benefits—for patients, providers, and society as a whole—are immense.

The current model is unsustainable, but the stories of patients like Richard, Gloria, and Derek remind me why we must push for change. By focusing on prevention, addressing root causes, and supporting patients holistically, we can create a system that truly prioritizes health over illness. It's not just a dream—it's a necessity for the future of healthcare in America.

℞ Dr. Crandall's Prescription for a New Healthcare Paradigm

✔ **Be Proactive in Your Healthcare.** Don't wait for symptoms to appear—schedule regular preventive care visits, screenings, and health assessments to stay ahead of potential issues.

✔ **Build a Partnership with Your Doctor.** Treat your healthcare provider as a partner in your well-being by asking questions, discussing concerns openly, and actively participating in decisions about your care.

✔ **Advocate for Your Health Needs.** If you feel your concerns aren't being addressed, seek second opinions or explore alternative providers to ensure your voice is heard and respected in your care.

✔ **Educate Yourself on Healthcare Options.** Learn about your insurance plan, available benefits, and local healthcare resources to make informed choices that align with your health and financial needs.

✔ **Focus on Long-Term Health Goals.** Shift your mindset from managing symptoms to improving overall health through sustainable lifestyle changes and preventive strategies.

✔ **Be Open to Integrative Care.** Explore complementary approaches like nutrition counseling, physical therapy, or stress management techniques as part of a holistic healthcare plan.

✔ **Encourage Preventive Practices in Your Circle.** Share knowledge about the importance of preventive care with family and friends to foster a culture of wellness within your community.

Resources

National Patient Advocate Foundation (NPAF)
Advocates making the healthcare system work for everyone, and offers support and education on how to navigate it for both patients and caregivers (https://www.npaf.org).

Patient Advocate Foundation
National non-profit organization that provides professional case management services to Americans with chronic, life-threatening and debilitating conditions (www.patientadvocate.org).

National Wellness Institute
A professional organization dedicated to advancing wellness across the United States. It offers a variety of resources, including webinars, certifications, and information on wellness programs and events (https://wellnessalliance.org).

Department of Health and Human Services (HHS) Prevention & Wellness
Resources on nutrition, fitness, immunizations, and screenings to help individuals maintain a healthy lifestyle and prevent chronic diseases (https://www.hhs.gov/programs/prevention-and-wellness).

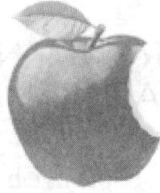

CHAPTER SIX

BUILDING HEALTHY COMMUNITIES

Health is not just an individual concern but also a community-wide challenge. The environments in which people live, work, and socialize significantly shape their health outcomes. While individual behaviors such as diet, exercise, and sleep are crucial to personal well-being, the broader context—urban design, access to resources, social support networks, and environmental factors—plays a vital role in determining whether individuals and communities can live healthy lives. Building healthy communities requires a multifaceted approach, addressing everything from food access and physical activity to social cohesion and environmental health.

This chapter explores how community design, public policies, and local initiatives can contribute to creating healthier neighborhoods. It highlights the importance of access to healthy food, opportunities for physical activity, green spaces, and strong social ties. Additionally, it delves into the role of community-led health initiatives and the policies that support or hinder the development of healthy environments.

THE ROLE OF ENVIRONMENT AND COMMUNITY IN SHAPING HEALTH OUTCOMES

The environments in which people live have a profound influence on health. The World Health Organization (WHO) estimates that up to 24% of global deaths are due to environmental factors, including air pollution, unsafe water, and poor housing conditions. In the United States, the impact of environmental factors is particularly pronounced in communities of color and low-income neighborhoods, where residents often experience higher rates of chronic diseases such as asthma, diabetes, and heart disease due to poor living conditions and limited access to healthcare.

One of the most significant determinants of health is *urban design*. The way cities and neighborhoods are built influences everything from physical activity levels to mental health. For example, communities that are walkable—those with sidewalks, bike lanes, parks, and pedestrian-friendly streets—encourage residents to engage in more physical activity. In contrast, neighborhoods that are designed for cars, with few sidewalks or safe crossings, discourage walking and biking, contributing to sedentary lifestyles.

Access to healthy food is another critical factor in shaping health outcomes. Many low-income neighborhoods are classified as "food deserts," meaning they lack access to affordable, nutritious food. Instead, residents often rely on convenience stores or fast food outlets that offer processed, unhealthy foods high in sugar, fat, and salt. This lack of access to healthy food contributes to higher rates of obesity, diabetes, and other diet-related illnesses in these communities.

Social cohesion and a sense of community also play a crucial role in health. People who feel connected to their neighbors and have strong social support networks are more likely to engage in healthy behaviors, such as exercising regularly, eating nutritious foods, and seeking medical care when needed. Conversely, social isolation is associated with poorer health outcomes, including higher rates of chronic disease, mental illness, and premature death.

Last, the *built environment* affects mental health as well. Research shows that access to green spaces, such as parks and nature reserves, can reduce stress, improve mood, and lower the risk of depression. In urban areas, where access to nature is often limited, creating more green spaces and promoting outdoor activities can significantly improve residents' mental well-being.

URBAN DESIGN AND HEALTH: HOW CITIES CAN PROMOTE WELL-BEING

Urban design has a direct impact on the health and well-being of residents. The layout of streets, the availability of public transportation, and the presence of parks and recreational spaces all influence whether people can easily engage in healthy activities. Cities that prioritize walkability, bikeability, and access to green spaces tend to have healthier populations.

Walkable neighborhoods are one of the most effective ways to promote physical activity. When residents can safely walk to schools, stores, and parks, they are more likely to incorporate walking into their daily routines. In contrast, neighborhoods without sidewalks, crosswalks, or street lighting make walking unsafe and unappealing, leading to more car use and sedentary behavior. Walkable cities also promote social interaction, as people are more likely to engage with their neighbors when walking through the community.

Bike-friendly infrastructure is another important element of healthy city design. Dedicated bike lanes, bike-sharing programs, and safe places to lock bicycles encourage more people to cycle, which not only is good for physical health but also reduces traffic congestion and air pollution. Cities like Copenhagen and Amsterdam, where biking is a primary mode of transportation, are often cited as models for how urban design can promote active living.

Access to parks and green spaces is equally essential for promoting health. Parks provide opportunities for physical activity, whether it's walking, jogging, playing sports, or simply enjoying nature. Green spaces also have mental health benefits, as spending time in nature has been shown to reduce stress and anxiety. In cities with limited green spaces, efforts to create more parks, community gardens, and outdoor recreation areas can significantly improve residents' quality of life.

Public transportation also plays a role in promoting health. Cities with reliable, affordable public transit systems make it easier for residents to access healthcare services, grocery stores, and other essential resources. Public transportation encourages more walking, as people often walk to and from bus stops or train stations. It also reduces air pollution by decreasing the number of cars on the road, which benefits respiratory health.

THE IMPORTANCE OF ACCESS TO HEALTHY FOODS

Access to healthy, affordable food is a fundamental component of building healthy communities. Unfortunately, many low-income neighborhoods in both urban and rural areas lack access to fresh fruits, vegetables, and other nutritious foods. Instead, these areas are dominated by convenience stores, fast food restaurants, and liquor stores, where unhealthy, processed foods are readily available.

Food deserts are a significant public health concern. Residents of food deserts are more likely to experience diet-related health problems, including obesity, diabetes, and heart disease. According to the USDA, approximately 19 million Americans live in food deserts, which are defined as areas where at least 33% of the population lives more than one mile from a grocery store in urban areas or more than 10 miles in rural areas.

Addressing food deserts requires a combination of policy changes and community-driven solutions. One approach is to *incentivize grocery stores* to open in underserved areas by offering tax breaks or subsidies. Programs like the Healthy Food Financing Initiative (HFFI) provide funding to help grocery stores and other healthy food retailers expand into low-income communities. Additionally, *mobile markets* and *farmers' markets* can bring fresh produce directly to neighborhoods that lack grocery stores.

Urban agriculture is another promising solution to the problem of food deserts. Community gardens, rooftop farms, and other urban farming initiatives allow residents to grow their own food, increasing access to fresh, healthy produce. Urban agriculture not only improves food security but also fosters a sense of community and provides educational opportunities around nutrition and sustainability.

Nutrition education programs are also crucial for promoting healthy eating. Many low-income families lack the knowledge or skills needed to prepare healthy meals on a budget. Cooking classes, nutrition workshops, and school-based programs can teach people how to make healthier food choices and prepare nutritious meals. Programs like SNAP-Ed (Supplemental Nutrition Assistance Program Education) provide low-income individuals with resources and education to help them make healthier choices within their budget.

THE ROLE OF SOCIAL COHESION IN BUILDING HEALTHY COMMUNITIES

A sense of community and strong social connections are essential for both mental and physical health. People who feel connected to their neighbors and have access to social support networks are more likely to engage in healthy behaviors and seek medical care when needed. Conversely, social isolation is linked to a range of negative health outcomes, including higher rates of chronic disease, mental illness, and premature death.

Social cohesion refers to the degree to which people in a community feel connected to one another. Communities with high levels of social cohesion tend to have lower crime rates, better health outcomes, and stronger social support networks. In these communities, neighbors look out for one another, share resources, and work together to solve problems.

Building social cohesion requires creating spaces and opportunities for people to connect. *Community centers, parks,* and *public gathering spaces* provide venues for social interaction. Events such as neighborhood festivals, block parties, and farmers' markets bring people together and foster a sense of belonging. Community-based organizations, churches, and schools can also play a role in strengthening social ties by organizing activities, support groups, and volunteer opportunities.

In addition to fostering social connections, *public safety* is an important component of social cohesion. People are more likely to engage with their community and participate in outdoor activities if they feel safe in their neighborhood. Efforts to reduce crime and improve public safety—such as community policing, neighborhood watch programs, and better street lighting—can encourage people to spend more time outdoors and interact with their neighbors.

Community-led initiatives are another powerful way to build social cohesion and improve health. When residents take ownership of the health and well-being of their community, they are more likely to make positive changes. For example, community health worker programs, in which local residents are trained to provide health education and support to their neighbors, have been successful in improving health outcomes in low-income communities. Similarly, neighborhood groups that organize clean-up efforts, beautification projects, and other community improvement activities can foster a sense of pride and connectedness.

POLICIES AND PROGRAMS THAT FOSTER HEALTHY COMMUNITIES

Government policies at the local, state, and federal levels play a crucial role in shaping the health of communities. Public policies that support affordable housing, access to healthcare, safe environments, and healthy food are essential for creating conditions in which people can thrive.

Affordable housing is a critical component of building healthy communities. Housing instability and poor living conditions are linked to a range of negative health outcomes, including higher rates of chronic disease, mental illness, and exposure to environmental hazards like mold and lead. Policies that promote affordable housing, such as inclusionary zoning, rent control, and housing subsidies, can help ensure that all residents have access to safe, stable housing.

Healthcare access is another key policy area. Expanding Medicaid and other public health insurance programs can help ensure that low-income residents have access to preventive care and treatment.

DR. CRANDALL'S AMERICA:
Building Healthy Communities

Over the years, I've seen firsthand how the environment people live in profoundly shapes their health. From the availability of nutritious food to the safety of their neighborhoods, the communities we live in either foster health or contribute to illness. As a doctor, I've been privileged to treat patients across a spectrum of environments, and their stories have taught me how vital it is to address the broader context of health, not just individual choices.

One patient who stands out is Patricia, a 35-year-old mother of two living in an urban neighborhood. Patricia struggled with obesity, high blood pressure, and stress-related anxiety. When I asked about her lifestyle, she shared how her environment was holding her back. "Doctor," she said, "there's no place for my kids to play safely, and I don't feel comfortable walking in my own neighborhood." Patricia's grocery store was a 30-minute bus ride away, and fast food was the easiest option for her family. Her story is one I've heard countless times—individuals wanting to make healthier choices but being constrained by the resources and safety of their surroundings.

I've also seen the stark contrast in communities that prioritize health. Early in my career, I worked in a suburban area where sidewalks were plentiful, parks were well-maintained, and farmers' markets were a regular fixture. The residents in these neighborhoods had lower rates of chronic illnesses and were more likely to engage in regular physical activity. I remember a patient, Carl, who told me, "Doctor, I love walking to the market every Saturday and picking out fresh produce." Carl's environment made it easy for him to make healthy choices, and it showed in his overall well-being.

But I've also seen the power of change, even in communities where the odds seemed stacked against health. In one town I worked in, a local coalition of churches and civic groups transformed an abandoned lot into a community garden. I'll never forget seeing the pride on a patient's face as she brought me fresh tomatoes and kale she had grown herself. "We never had anything like this before," she said. The garden not only provided fresh produce to a food desert but also created a sense of connection and hope among residents.

However, not every effort succeeds. In another underserved neighborhood, a plan to open a community center with fitness programs and after-school activities fell through due to lack of funding. The disappointment among residents was palpable. One patient, a young father named Eric, told me, "We really thought this could make a difference." His frustration was a reminder of how often systemic barriers—like funding shortages and bureaucratic hurdles—undermine initiatives that could genuinely improve community health.

These stories have shown me that while individual effort is important, the health of a community depends on collective action. Building healthier communities means addressing the root causes of poor health, from food deserts to unsafe streets. It requires collaboration among healthcare providers, local governments, businesses, and residents. I've seen how effective this collaboration can be, but I've also seen how challenging it is to achieve without the necessary support and resources.

Despite the challenges, I remain hopeful. I've seen communities rally to create walking trails, farmers' markets, and fitness programs. I've seen schools incorporate healthier meals and physical activity into their curricula. And I've seen how even small changes—like adding a few streetlights or opening a community gym— can have a ripple effect on public health.

As a doctor, I can prescribe medications and offer advice, but I know that true health requires more than what happens in an exam room. It requires environments that support healthy living and communities that prioritize well-being. The patients I've treated and the neighborhoods I've worked in have reinforced my belief that creating healthier communities is both a moral imperative and a practical necessity. By addressing the systemic factors that shape health, we can build a future where everyone has the opportunity to thrive.

R℞ Dr. Crandall's Prescription for Building Healthy Communities

✔ **Advocate for Safe and Walkable Neighborhoods.** Support local initiatives to improve sidewalks, bike lanes, and parks to encourage more active lifestyles.

✔ **Participate in Community Health Programs.** Engage in local health initiatives, such as fitness groups, farmers' markets, or wellness workshops, to foster a culture of well-being.

✔ **Encourage Schools to Implement Healthier Policies.** Work with local schools to improve access to nutritious meals, physical education, and mental health resources for children.

✔ **Support Local Businesses that Promote Health.** Choose grocery stores, restaurants, and organizations that prioritize fresh, whole foods and sustainable products.

✔ **Organize or Join Volunteer Efforts for Public Health.** Help create or participate in initiatives like clean-up drives, community gardens, or free health screenings to improve local environments.

✔ **Promote Mental Health Awareness in Your Community.** Encourage open discussions about mental well-being, advocate for accessible counseling services, and reduce stigma around seeking help.

✔ **Strengthen Social Connections.** Build relationships with neighbors, support networks, and local groups to create a healthier and more connected community.

Resources

Families USA
A leading, nonprofit, nonpartisan consumer health advocacy organization that has played a pivotal role in shaping healthcare legislation and policy (https://www.familiesusa.org).

Alliance for Health Policy
A nonpartisan, nonprofit organization is committed to enhancing understanding of health policy issues among policymakers and the public, facilitating informed discussions on healthcare reforms (https://www.allhealthpolicy.org).

USDA Local Food Directory
A guide to finding farmers markets across the country, you can just plug in the name of your city and/or your zip code (www .usdalocalfoodportal.com).

SAFE Project ("Guide to Building Your SAFE Community")
Offers a structured approach to mobilizing community resources against substance abuse and related issues (https://www.safeproject .us).

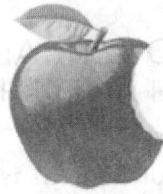

CHAPTER SEVEN

FIXING THE FOOD SYSTEM

The American food system is both a marvel of modern production and distribution and a source of deep concern for its negative impacts on health, the environment, and social equity. On the one hand, the U.S. food industry is incredibly efficient, producing a vast array of foods and making them available across the country at relatively low prices. On the other hand, this same system promotes the consumption of unhealthy, processed foods, perpetuates environmental degradation, and exacerbates food insecurity for millions of Americans.

The growing rates of obesity, diabetes, and other diet-related diseases highlight the need for change in how food is produced, distributed, and consumed. At the same time, issues like food deserts, the environmental impacts of industrial agriculture, and the unethical treatment of workers within the food supply chain demand attention. This chapter explores how the food system has contributed to public health challenges and what can be done to fix it. By addressing issues at the intersection of food, health, and sustainability, we can create a food system that nourishes people, protects the planet, and promotes social equity.

THE IMPACT OF INDUSTRIAL AGRICULTURE ON PUBLIC HEALTH AND THE ENVIRONMENT

The modern American food system is dominated by industrial agriculture, a highly mechanized and large-scale approach to farming that prioritizes efficiency and profit over environmental sustainability and human health. This model has successfully increased food production, making calories cheap and abundant. However, it has come at a high cost to both public health and the environment.

One of the most pressing health concerns related to industrial agriculture is the *overproduction of cheap, calorie-dense, nutrient-poor foods*. Corn, soy, and wheat—heavily subsidized by government policies—are the dominant crops in the United States, and they form the foundation of many processed foods. Corn and soy, in particular, are used to produce high-fructose corn syrup and hydrogenated oils, which are common ingredients in junk food and are linked to obesity, heart disease, and other chronic conditions. These cheap ingredients have made it easier for food manufacturers to produce and market processed snacks, sugary drinks, and fast food, which are now staples in the American diet.

In addition to its impact on public health, industrial agriculture is one of the leading contributors to *environmental degradation*. The use of synthetic fertilizers and pesticides in large-scale farming has polluted waterways, destroyed biodiversity, and depleted soil health. Industrial agriculture is also a significant driver of climate change, as it relies heavily on fossil fuels for machinery, transportation, and the production of fertilizers. Livestock production, particularly beef, contributes significantly to greenhouse gas emissions, with cattle farming producing large amounts of methane, a potent greenhouse gas.

The environmental impacts of industrial agriculture are not limited to climate change. The destruction of ecosystems through deforestation and monoculture farming (the practice of planting the same crop year after year) has led to the loss of biodiversity. Soil degradation is another major issue, as industrial farming practices strip the soil of nutrients, making it less fertile and more dependent on chemical inputs. This cycle of environmental harm perpetuates a system that is unsustainable in the long term.

FOOD DESERTS AND FOOD INSECURITY

One of the most glaring inequalities in the American food system is the existence of *food deserts*. Food deserts are most commonly found in low-income urban and rural areas, where there are few grocery stores or supermarkets. Instead, residents of these areas often rely on convenience stores and fast food outlets, which offer mostly processed, unhealthy foods. The lack of access to fresh fruits, vegetables, and whole grains in food deserts contributes to poor diet quality and higher rates of diet-related diseases like obesity, diabetes, and hypertension.

The USDA defines food deserts as areas where at least 500 people, or 33% of the population, live more than one mile away from a grocery store in urban areas or more than 10 miles away in rural areas. The presence of food deserts disproportionately affects communities of color and low-income households, exacerbating existing health disparities. Food insecurity, the condition of not having reliable access to enough nutritious food, is another major issue. According to the USDA, more than 38 million people in the United States, including 12 million children, were food insecure in 2020.

Food insecurity is closely linked to health problems. Individuals and families who are food insecure are more likely to suffer from chronic diseases due to the poor quality of the foods they can afford or access. This can create a vicious cycle, as poor health outcomes can lead to medical expenses that further strain household budgets, making it even more difficult to afford nutritious food.

Solving the problem of food deserts and food insecurity requires systemic changes in how food is produced, distributed, and priced. Government programs such as the Supplemental Nutrition Assistance Program (SNAP) and Women, Infants, and Children (WIC) provide essential support to low-income households, but more can be done to ensure that healthy, fresh foods are available and affordable in all communities.

THE RISE OF ORGANIC, LOCAL, AND REGENERATIVE FARMING

In response to the negative impacts of industrial agriculture, there has been a growing movement toward *organic, local,* and *regenerative farming* practices. These alternative farming systems prioritize environmental sustainability, animal welfare, and human health. While still a small portion of the overall food system, these movements are gaining traction as consumers become more aware of the environmental and health consequences of industrial food production.

Organic farming avoids the use of synthetic pesticides and fertilizers, instead relying on natural methods to manage pests and improve soil fertility. Organic farmers use practices such as crop rotation, composting, and biological pest control to grow food in ways that are healthier for both people and the planet. Organic foods are free from harmful chemicals, which can reduce the risk of exposure to toxins and improve overall health outcomes for consumers. Moreover, organic farming promotes biodiversity and protects ecosystems by avoiding the destructive practices associated with industrial agriculture.

Local food systems are another important alternative to industrial agriculture. Local food systems prioritize the production and consumption of food within a specific geographic area, reducing the carbon footprint associated with transporting food long distances.

Farmers' markets, community-supported agriculture (CSA) programs, and farm-to-table restaurants have grown in popularity as more consumers seek out fresh, local foods that support small farmers and reduce environmental impact. By purchasing locally grown foods, consumers can support their local economies, strengthen community ties, and ensure that their food is produced in ways that align with their values.

Regenerative agriculture goes a step further by not only avoiding environmental harm but actively working to restore ecosystems. Regenerative farming practices, such as cover cropping, rotational grazing, and agroforestry, improve soil health, increase biodiversity, and sequester carbon from the atmosphere. This approach to farming is seen as a potential solution to both food production and climate change, as it seeks to create a sustainable, closed-loop system that mimics natural ecosystems. Regenerative agriculture offers a hopeful vision for the future of farming, one that prioritizes ecological balance and long-term sustainability.

While organic, local, and regenerative farming represent promising alternatives to industrial agriculture, they face significant challenges. These systems are often more labor-intensive and expensive to implement, which can drive up the cost of food for consumers. Additionally, they currently make up only a small fraction of the overall food supply, meaning that their impact is still limited. To truly transform the food system, these practices will need to be scaled up and supported by both government policies and consumer demand.

GOVERNMENT POLICIES AND THE FOOD SYSTEM

Government policies play a significant role in shaping the American food system, influencing everything from the types of crops that are grown to the prices consumers pay at the grocery store. Historically,

U.S. agricultural policies have favored the production of commodity crops like corn, soy, and wheat, which are used to produce processed foods and animal feed. These crops receive the majority of federal subsidies, making them cheap to produce and purchase. In contrast, fruits, vegetables, and other specialty crops receive far less government support, contributing to the higher prices of healthy foods relative to unhealthy, processed options.

Farm subsidies are one of the most influential aspects of U.S. food policy. These subsidies were originally designed during the Great Depression to support struggling farmers and stabilize food prices. However, over time, they have become a mechanism for promoting the overproduction of certain crops, particularly corn and soy, which are used to make cheap processed foods and feed for livestock. This overproduction has led to a glut of unhealthy, calorie-dense foods that are readily available in the American diet.

Reforming farm subsidies is a critical step in fixing the food system. By shifting subsidies away from commodity crops and toward the production of fruits, vegetables, and other healthy foods, the government can help make nutritious food more affordable and accessible. Additionally, policies that support small and mid-sized farms, rather than large agribusinesses, can promote more sustainable and equitable food production.

Food labeling laws are another important area of policy that can influence consumer behavior and promote healthier eating. Clear, transparent labeling of ingredients, nutritional content, and food origin can help consumers make more informed choices. For example, labels that indicate whether a product contains genetically modified organisms (GMOs) or was produced using organic methods allow consumers to align their food purchases with their values. Additionally, front-of-package labels that clearly indicate the levels of sugar, fat, and sodium in a product can help consumers make healthier choices, particularly when it comes to processed foods.

Food assistance programs such as SNAP and WIC are essential for ensuring that low-income households have access to nutritious food.

However, these programs can be improved to better promote healthy eating. For example, increasing the value of SNAP benefits when used to purchase fruits and vegetables can incentivize healthier food choices. Programs like the Double Up Food Bucks initiative, which matches SNAP dollars spent on fresh produce, have shown promising results in improving diet quality among low-income families.

THE ROLE OF SCHOOLS AND INSTITUTIONS IN SHAPING FOOD HABITS

Schools and other institutions play a crucial role in shaping the food habits of children and adults alike. The foods served in school cafeterias, hospitals, prisons, and government buildings have a direct impact on the health of the people who consume them, as well as on the broader food system.

School lunch programs are one of the most important avenues for improving children's health and addressing diet-related diseases. For many children, especially those from low-income families, school meals are a primary source of nutrition. Unfortunately, the quality of these meals has often been lacking, with processed foods high in fat, sugar, and sodium dominating school menus. However, recent reforms, such as the Healthy, Hunger-Free Kids Act of 2010, have made strides in improving the nutritional quality of school meals by setting stricter standards for the inclusion of fruits, vegetables, whole grains, and lean proteins.

Expanding the availability of *farm-to-school programs*, which connect schools with local farmers to provide fresh, locally grown foods in cafeterias, is another effective way to improve the quality of school meals. These programs not only provide healthier food options for students but also support local farmers and educate children about where their food comes from. School gardens, nutrition education programs, and cooking classes can also help foster healthy eating habits that last a lifetime.

Beyond schools, other institutions, like hospitals and workplaces, can promote healthier food environments by offering nutritious meal options and encouraging healthy eating. *Hospital food* has long been criticized for being unhealthy and unappetizing, but some healthcare institutions are now leading the way in promoting healthier food choices. For example, some hospitals have introduced *food pharmacies*, where patients with diet-related illnesses can receive fresh produce and healthy meal kits as part of their treatment plans. These programs not only improve patient health but also send a powerful message about the importance of food in medicine.

THE PATH FORWARD: A HEALTHIER, MORE SUSTAINABLE FOOD SYSTEM

Fixing the American food system requires a multi-pronged approach that addresses public health, environmental sustainability, and social equity. While the challenges are significant, there are numerous opportunities to create a food system that nourishes both people and the planet.

- **Supporting small and sustainable farms** is essential for promoting biodiversity, reducing environmental harm, and improving food quality. Policies that provide financial incentives for organic, local, and regenerative farming practices can help scale up these alternatives to industrial agriculture.
- **Expanding access to healthy foods** through government programs, urban agriculture, and improved food distribution networks can reduce food deserts and food insecurity. Making healthy food more affordable and accessible to all Americans is crucial for improving public health outcomes.
- **Promoting transparency and education** in the food system through better food labeling, nutrition education in schools, and public awareness campaigns can help consumers make healthier, more informed choices.

- **Reforming food policies** to prioritize health and sustainability over profit is necessary for creating long-term change. Shifting subsidies, improving food assistance programs, and enacting stronger regulations on processed foods will be key to fixing the food system.

By taking these steps, we can create a food system that supports healthy eating, protects the environment, and promotes social justice, ultimately leading to a healthier and more sustainable future for all.

DR. CRANDALL'S AMERICA:
Fixing the Food System

Throughout my career, I have seen how deeply the food system impacts my patients' health. The way food is produced, marketed, and distributed in America has created a landscape where unhealthy choices are often the most accessible and affordable. As a doctor, I've witnessed the devastating consequences of this reality, but I've also seen the potential for change when communities and individuals take steps to fix the broken food system.

One patient who stands out is Angela, a 40-year-old single mother of three who came to me struggling with obesity and type 2 diabetes. Angela worked two jobs and relied on processed, fast food to feed her family because it was cheap and convenient. She told me, "Doctor, I know it's not good for us, but it's all I can afford, and I don't have time to cook." Her story is one I hear over and over again—a reflection of how the food system fails so many families by making unhealthy options the easiest choice.

Angela's turning point came when her local community center started offering free cooking classes and distributing fresh produce through a partnership with a nearby farm. With some guidance, Angela began preparing simple, nutritious meals for her family. Over the next year, she lost weight, improved her blood sugar levels, and, most importantly, felt empowered to take control of her family's health. "I didn't think it was possible," she told me, "but now my kids even prefer the home-cooked meals." Her story gives me hope that change is possible, but it also underscores how much support is needed to overcome the systemic barriers so many people face.

Not all stories are as uplifting. I recall a young man named Derek who was in his early thirties but already suffering from high cholesterol, hypertension, and prediabetes. Derek lived in a food desert, where the closest grocery store was miles away, and the only nearby food options were fast-food restaurants and convenience stores. "I'd love to eat healthier," he told me, "but there's nowhere to buy fresh vegetables around here." Derek's situation highlights the stark inequities in food access that are rampant in both rural and urban areas across America.

As a medical missionary, I've also seen the stark contrast between traditional diets and the influence of the globalized food system. In one village in Africa, I worked with communities who thrived on diets of locally grown fruits, vegetables, and whole grains. The rates of obesity, diabetes, and heart disease were almost nonexistent. But even in these remote areas, the encroachment of processed, sugary, and packaged foods was starting to take hold. It was a stark reminder of how the problems created by industrialized food systems are not confined to America—they're spreading worldwide.

I've also been inspired by grassroots efforts to fix the food system. In one community I worked in, a group of local farmers partnered with schools to provide fresh produce for school lunches. The program didn't just improve the nutritional quality of meals; it also taught children about where their food came from and the importance of eating fresh, whole foods. One parent told me, "My daughter never liked vegetables before, but now she's asking me to buy kale!" Programs like this remind me that education and access can go hand in hand to create lasting change.

But I've also seen the challenges these programs face. One local farmers' market I visited struggled to stay open because of a lack of funding and support. The market was a lifeline for many low-income families who relied on it for fresh produce. Its closure was a harsh reminder of how fragile these efforts can be without systemic backing from governments and policymakers.

These stories have shaped my belief that fixing the food system is one of the most critical steps we can take to improve public health. It's not just about individual choices—it's about creating a system where healthy options are accessible, affordable, and sustainable for everyone. Whether it's through policy changes, community initiatives, or partnerships with local farmers, we need a collective effort to make this happen.

The patients I've treated and the communities I've worked in have shown me both the depth of the problem and the incredible potential for change. With the right support and resources, we can create a food system that nourishes rather than harms—and in doing so, we can give everyone the opportunity to lead healthier, fuller lives.

R̷X Dr. Crandall's Prescription for Fixing the Food System

✔ **Support Local and Regenerative Farming.** Buy from local farmers' markets or community-supported agriculture (CSA) programs to promote sustainable, ethical food production.

✔ **Advocate for Transparent Food Labeling.** Push for clearer ingredient lists and labeling on processed foods to make informed choices about what goes into your body.

✔ **Reduce Reliance on Ultra-Processed Foods.** Prioritize whole foods over packaged, highly processed options that contribute to obesity, inflammation, and chronic disease.

✔ **Grow Your Own Food When Possible.** Even small-scale gardening, such as growing herbs or vegetables in pots, can increase access to fresh, nutritious foods.

✔ **Encourage Healthy Food Options in Schools and Workplaces.** Advocate for nutritious meal programs in schools and workplace cafeterias to improve access to healthier choices.

✔ **Be Aware of Corporate Influence on Food Policy.** Stay informed about how large food corporations shape regulations and work to support policies that prioritize health over profit.

✔ **Minimize Food Waste.** Plan meals, store food properly, and repurpose leftovers to reduce waste and make the most of available resources.

Resources

Farmers Market Coalition (FMC)
Provides resources and a searchable database of farmers' markets by state (https://farmersmarketcoalition.org).

LocalHarvest

A locator to find farmers' markets, family farms, organic food businesses, and other local food sources in your area (https://www .localharvest.org).

National Farmers Market Directory

A searchable list of farmers' markets nationwide so you can find one in your community (https://nfmd.org).

Feeding America

Feeding America is the largest hunger-relief organization in the United States that works to reduce food waste by redistributing surplus food to food banks, shelters, and community organizations. It operates over 200 food banks across the country (https://www .feedingamerica.org).

School Nutrition Association (SNA)

Advocates policies that improve the quality of school meals (https:// schoolnutrition.org).

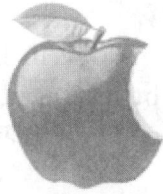

CHAPTER EIGHT

THE ROLE OF TECHNOLOGY IN HEALTH

As technology continues to evolve at an unprecedented pace, its impact on health and healthcare has been transformative. From fitness trackers and health apps that monitor personal health metrics to telemedicine platforms that expand access to care, technology has revolutionized how people manage their health and interact with healthcare systems. The integration of artificial intelligence (AI), big data analytics, and wearable devices has created opportunities for early disease detection, personalized treatment, and improved patient outcomes. However, this growing reliance on digital health tools also raises important questions about privacy, equity, and the potential over-reliance on technology at the expense of traditional healthcare practices.

In this chapter, we will explore how digital health tools are transforming the way people approach their health, the benefits and challenges of wearable technology, and the role of AI and big data in predicting and preventing disease. Additionally, we will examine the ethical considerations surrounding privacy, data security, and the digital divide. Ultimately, the goal is to understand both the potential and the limitations of technology in healthcare and to explore how these innovations can be leveraged to create a more efficient, accessible, and patient-centered healthcare system.

HOW DIGITAL HEALTH TOOLS ARE TRANSFORMING HEALTHCARE

The rise of *digital health tools*—including mobile apps, wearable devices, telemedicine platforms, and online patient portals—has shifted the landscape of healthcare. These tools empower individuals to take more control of their health by providing real-time data, facilitating remote consultations, and improving communication between patients and healthcare providers. Digital health tools have the potential to democratize healthcare by making it more accessible and personalized, particularly for those who live in remote areas or face barriers to accessing traditional healthcare services.

One of the most significant advances in digital health is the *telemedicine* revolution. Telemedicine, or the use of digital communication technologies to provide healthcare remotely, has gained widespread adoption, particularly during the COVID-19 pandemic. With telemedicine, patients can consult with doctors, therapists, and specialists from the comfort of their own homes, reducing the need for in-person visits and making healthcare more convenient. This has been particularly beneficial for individuals with mobility issues, those living in rural areas with limited access to healthcare, and people seeking mental health services, where face-to-face interactions are not always necessary.

Telemedicine also offers the potential to reduce *healthcare disparities* by expanding access to care for underserved populations. For example, rural residents who may have to travel long distances to see a specialist can now consult with healthcare providers virtually, improving their access to care. Similarly, individuals with chronic conditions can use telemedicine to manage their health more effectively by having regular check-ins with their healthcare team without the inconvenience of frequent office visits.

In addition to telemedicine, *wearable health devices* such as fitness trackers, smartwatches, and connected health monitors have become increasingly popular. These devices allow individuals to track various health metrics, such as heart rate, sleep patterns, physical activity, and even blood glucose levels for people with diabetes. By providing users with real-time data about their health, wearable devices encourage people to engage in healthier behaviors, such as exercising more, sleeping better, and managing stress levels.

Moreover, wearable devices can serve as early warning systems for detecting health issues. For example, smartwatches equipped with electrocardiogram (ECG) sensors can detect irregular heartbeats, potentially alerting users to the risk of atrial fibrillation, a condition that increases the risk of stroke. Similarly, wearable devices can monitor sleep patterns and detect sleep apnea, a condition that is linked to cardiovascular disease, diabetes, and other health problems. These early detection capabilities can prompt users to seek medical attention before a condition becomes more serious, leading to better health outcomes.

Mobile health apps have also proliferated, offering a wide range of services, from tracking diet and exercise to managing chronic conditions like diabetes or asthma. Apps like MyFitnessPal and Lose It! help users log their meals and track their calorie intake, while others, like Headspace and Calm, offer guided meditation and mindfulness practices to reduce stress and improve mental health. Apps that provide medication reminders, such as Medisafe, can help patients manage complex medication regimens, improving adherence to prescribed treatments and reducing the risk of complications.

THE BENEFITS AND PITFALLS OF WEARABLE TECHNOLOGY

Wearable technology has immense potential to improve health outcomes by encouraging healthier behaviors and enabling early detection of medical conditions. However, the widespread use of these devices also comes with certain challenges and limitations.

One of the primary benefits of *wearable technology* is its ability to engage individuals in their own health management. Many people find that tracking their daily steps, heart rate, or sleep patterns motivates them to make healthier choices, such as being more active or getting more rest. This sense of accountability can be particularly helpful for individuals who are trying to lose weight, manage a chronic condition, or improve their overall fitness.

In addition, wearables provide *continuous health monitoring*, which can offer a more comprehensive picture of a person's health than traditional, episodic check-ups with a doctor. For example, instead of relying on blood pressure readings taken only during office visits, wearable devices can track blood pressure throughout the day, providing more accurate data and helping doctors identify trends or patterns that may indicate a health issue. Continuous monitoring is especially valuable for individuals with chronic conditions such as heart disease, diabetes, or hypertension, where frequent tracking of health metrics is essential for effective management.

However, wearable technology is not without its pitfalls. One of the primary concerns is *data accuracy*. While wearable devices are useful for tracking general trends in activity levels or heart rate, they may not always provide precise medical data. For example, studies have shown that the calorie counts provided by fitness trackers can vary widely in accuracy, leading to potential misinformation about energy expenditure. Similarly, the ECG functions of smartwatches are not a replacement for clinical tests performed by healthcare professionals. Inaccurate data can lead users to make inappropriate decisions about their health, such as overestimating their level of fitness or ignoring symptoms that may require medical attention.

Another challenge is *user engagement*. While many people are enthusiastic about their wearables when they first start using them, studies have shown that long-term engagement often declines.

People may lose interest in tracking their health metrics over time, especially if they do not see immediate results. Additionally, the constant monitoring and feedback provided by wearable devices can sometimes lead to *unhealthy obsessions* with health data, particularly for individuals prone to anxiety or perfectionism. In these cases, wearables may exacerbate stress rather than improve well-being.

Privacy concerns are also a major issue with wearable technology. Devices like fitness trackers and smartwatches collect vast amounts of personal health data, which is often stored in the cloud or shared with third-party companies. This raises questions about who has access to this data, how it is being used, and how secure it is. In the event of a data breach, sensitive health information could be exposed, leading to potential privacy violations. Moreover, as more employers and insurance companies offer incentives for using wearables, there is a risk that this data could be used to penalize individuals based on their health behaviors or conditions.

THE ROLE OF ARTIFICIAL INTELLIGENCE AND BIG DATA IN HEALTH

One of the most exciting developments in healthcare is the increasing use of *artificial intelligence (AI)* and *big data analytics* to predict, prevent, and treat disease. AI and big data have the potential to revolutionize healthcare by making it more personalized, efficient, and effective.

AI can process vast amounts of health data quickly and accurately, allowing for the development of predictive models that can identify individuals at risk for certain conditions before symptoms appear. For example, AI algorithms can analyze electronic health records (EHRs) to identify patterns and correlations that may not be immediately apparent to human doctors. This can help detect early signs of diseases like cancer or heart disease, allowing for earlier interventions and improving patient outcomes.

In addition to early detection, AI is being used to develop *personalized treatment plans*. By analyzing a patient's genetic information, lifestyle, and medical history, AI can recommend the most effective treatments for that individual. This is particularly valuable in fields like oncology, where personalized medicine is becoming increasingly important. For example, AI can analyze the genetic mutations of a cancer tumor and suggest targeted therapies that are more likely to be effective for that specific patient, rather than relying on a one-size-fits-all approach.

Big data also plays a crucial role in public health. By analyzing large datasets from sources like hospital records, wearable devices, and social media, public health officials can gain insights into the spread of diseases, the effectiveness of treatments, and the social determinants of health. For example, during the COVID-19 pandemic, big data was used to track infection rates, identify hotspots, and predict the impact of public health interventions. This allowed policymakers to make more informed decisions and allocate resources more effectively.

However, the use of AI and big data in healthcare also raises important ethical concerns. One of the primary concerns is *bias* in AI algorithms. If the data used to train AI models is biased—such as underrepresenting certain racial or ethnic groups—the resulting predictions and recommendations may be biased as well. This could lead to unequal treatment and exacerbate existing health disparities. Ensuring that AI models are trained on diverse datasets and regularly audited for bias is essential for creating fair and equitable healthcare systems.

Another concern is *data privacy*. As more health data is collected and shared, the risk of data breaches and unauthorized access increases. Protecting patient data is critical to maintaining trust in digital health technologies. Strict regulations, such as the Health Insurance Portability and Accountability Act (HIPAA), govern the use of health data in the United States, but as technology evolves, there may be a need for updated regulations to address new privacy challenges.

ETHICAL CONSIDERATIONS: PRIVACY, EQUITY, AND THE DIGITAL DIVIDE

The increasing reliance on technology in healthcare raises important *ethical considerations* that must be addressed to ensure that these innovations benefit everyone.

Privacy is one of the most pressing concerns. As more personal health data is collected through wearable devices, mobile apps, and AI-driven tools, individuals may worry about how their data is being used and who has access to it. Ensuring that health data is protected and that individuals have control over how their data is shared is essential. Healthcare providers, app developers, and technology companies must prioritize data security and transparency to maintain trust.

Equity is another critical issue. While digital health tools have the potential to improve access to care, they also risk widening the gap between those who have access to technology and those who do not. This is known as the *digital divide*. Individuals in low-income communities, older adults, and people living in rural areas may not have the same access to smartphones, computers, or reliable internet connections as others, making it more difficult for them to benefit from telemedicine or wearable devices. Addressing the digital divide requires investment in infrastructure, affordable internet access, and digital literacy programs to ensure that everyone can take advantage of the benefits of health technology.

Additionally, there is a risk that *technology could replace traditional care*, particularly in situations where human interaction is important. While telemedicine is a convenient option for many patients, it should not completely replace in-person visits, especially for those with complex medical conditions that require physical exams or hands-on treatment. Ensuring that technology complements, rather than replaces, human care is essential for maintaining the quality and compassion of healthcare services.

THE FUTURE OF HEALTH TECHNOLOGY

As technology continues to evolve, the future of healthcare looks increasingly digital. *Wearable devices* will become more sophisticated, offering deeper insights into health metrics and integrating seamlessly with healthcare systems. *AI and big data* will continue to drive advances in personalized medicine and disease prevention, making healthcare more predictive and proactive.

In the future, *precision medicine* will likely play a more prominent role in healthcare, with treatments tailored to an individual's genetic makeup, environment, and lifestyle. The integration of *genomics* and *AI* will allow doctors to prescribe treatments that are highly personalized, improving outcomes and reducing side effects.

However, as technology becomes more ingrained in healthcare, there will need to be a continued focus on *ethical considerations*, including privacy, equity, and the role of human interaction in care. Ensuring that technological innovations benefit everyone, rather than just those with the resources to access them, will be key to creating a more equitable healthcare system.

CONCLUSION: TECHNOLOGY AS A TOOL FOR HEALTH, NOT A REPLACEMENT FOR CARE

The role of technology in health is undeniably transformative, offering opportunities for improved access, personalized care, and early detection of diseases. From wearable devices that track health metrics to AI that predicts medical outcomes, the integration of technology has the potential to make healthcare more efficient and effective.

However, technology should be viewed as a tool for enhancing care, not replacing it. While digital health tools offer convenience and new insights, they cannot substitute for the compassion and expertise of healthcare professionals. Moreover, the widespread adoption of health technology must be accompanied by efforts to address privacy concerns, reduce health disparities, and ensure that technology complements human care.

By striking the right balance between technology and traditional healthcare practices, we can create a system that delivers better health outcomes for all, regardless of socioeconomic status, geographic location, or technological literacy.

DR. CRANDALL'S AMERICA:
The Role of Technology in Health

Over the years, I've witnessed the growing influence of technology in medicine—both its remarkable potential to improve lives and the challenges it brings. From telemedicine to wearable devices, technology has transformed how we deliver and monitor healthcare. Yet, my experiences have also shown me that not all patients benefit equally, and technological advancements sometimes exacerbate existing disparities.

One memorable patient was Tom, a 55-year-old man recovering from a heart attack. After his discharge, we equipped him with a wearable device to monitor his heart rate, activity levels, and sleep patterns. For Tom, this technology was life-changing. He became engaged in his own recovery, using the data to adjust his daily routines and improve his lifestyle. "It's like having you in my pocket, Doc," he joked during a follow-up visit. Tom's case highlights how technology can empower patients to take an active role in their health, transforming outcomes in the process.

But not every story is as seamless. I recall a young mother, Jasmine, who had been diagnosed with hypertension during her pregnancy. I recommended a remote monitoring system that would allow her to track her blood pressure at home. However, she lacked reliable internet access and struggled to navigate the technology. "I feel like this is more stress than help," she told me. Jasmine's case underscored a hard truth: While technology has the power to improve care, it can also create new barriers for patients who lack access to digital tools or the skills to use them.

As a doctor working in underserved communities, I've often seen how the digital divide prevents patients from reaping the benefits of health technology. In one rural town I visited, telemedicine was touted as a solution to the shortage of specialists, but many residents didn't have broadband internet or smartphones. One elderly patient, George, shared his frustration: "They say I can see a doctor on the computer, but I don't even know how to turn the thing on." For George and many like him, the promise of telemedicine remained out of reach.

Despite these challenges, I've also seen technology used creatively to bridge gaps. In a community health program I worked with, a team of volunteers provided free classes to teach patients how to use digital health tools, from blood pressure cuffs to telehealth apps. I'll never forget seeing the joy on a patient's face when she successfully completed her first telemedicine appointment. "I didn't think I could do this," she said. Initiatives like this remind me that with the right support, technology can empower even the most underserved populations.

One of the most exciting innovations I've encountered is the use of artificial intelligence (AI) in diagnosing conditions. I worked on a project where AI algorithms analyzed patient data to identify those at high risk for heart disease. The results were astonishing—we identified patients who might have otherwise slipped through the cracks and provided them with preventive care. However, I also saw the limitations: some patients were wary of technology making decisions about their health, and there was always the question of how to interpret and act on the vast amounts of data these tools generate.

What I've learned through these experiences is that while technology has enormous potential to improve health, it's not a silver bullet. It must be implemented thoughtfully, with a focus on equity and accessibility. Patients like Tom thrive with these tools, but patients like Jasmine and George remind me that technology alone isn't enough—it must be paired with education, infrastructure, and human connection.

Technology in healthcare is a powerful tool, but it's just that—a tool. It's how we use it, and for whom, that determines its impact. My patients have shown me that while technology can make incredible things possible, it must be integrated with compassion, understanding, and a commitment to bridging gaps. When we get that balance right, the possibilities for improving health outcomes are limitless.

℞ Dr. Crandall's Prescription for Maximizing the Role of Technology in Health

✔ **Leverage Wearable Devices for Accountability.** Use fitness trackers, smartwatches, or health apps to monitor daily activity, sleep, and other health metrics, fostering greater self-awareness and accountability.

✔ **Explore Telemedicine Options.** Take advantage of virtual healthcare appointments for convenience and access to specialists, particularly if location or time constraints are barriers.

✔ **Use Health Apps for Education and Support.** Download reputable apps to learn about nutrition, mental health, fitness, or chronic disease management, empowering yourself with actionable knowledge.

✔ **Set Digital Health Reminders.** Use technology to schedule reminders for medications, hydration, or stretching breaks, integrating health-focused habits into daily routines.

✔ **Engage in Online Health Communities.** Join virtual support groups or forums focused on wellness, chronic conditions, or fitness goals to find inspiration and share experiences with others on similar journeys.

✔ **Track Progress Over Time.** Use digital tools to chart improvements in key health areas, such as blood pressure, weight, or fitness levels, helping you stay motivated and informed.

✔ **Be Mindful of Privacy and Credibility.** Research and choose technology solutions with strong data protection policies and consult evidence-based sources to ensure the accuracy of information and tools.

Resources

Michael Miller. *Using Artificial Intelligence: Absolute Beginner's Guide*, 1st Edition. Que Publishing, 2024. Available through major booksellers and AARP, which offers a member's discount. Check the AARP member's website.

Dr. Anjum Ahmed and Dr. Po Hao-Chen, contributor. *AI in Healthcare: From Basics to Breakthroughs, Your Guide to the Heart of Healthcare's Future*, 2nd Edition, independently published, 2024.

Telehealth.HHS.gov (U.S. Department of Health and Human Services) Covers topics including what telehealth is, how to prepare for virtual visits, and tips for using technology (https://telehealth.hhs.gov).

HealthIT.gov
What You Can Do to Protect Your Health Information. A guide to steps for safeguarding your health data, such as reviewing privacy policies of online health platforms and utilizing strong passwords (https://telehealth.hhs.gov).

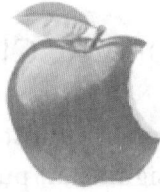

CHAPTER NINE

COMBATING HEALTH MISINFORMATION: RETHINKING THE SAFETY OF VACCINES

T he conversation around vaccines has become a polarizing topic in public health, with strong narratives supporting the idea that "all vaccines are safe." However, growing evidence and public concern suggest that this blanket statement may not always reflect the complex reality of vaccine safety. While vaccines have undoubtedly played a critical role in reducing the spread of infectious diseases and saving lives, it is important to acknowledge that not all vaccines are without risks. In recent years, reports of adverse effects and long-term health consequences have raised questions about the safety of certain vaccines for both children and adults.

This chapter delves into the concerns surrounding vaccine safety, exploring potential risks that have been reported, including severe allergic reactions, autoimmune disorders, and neurological effects. By addressing these issues openly, we aim to provide a more nuanced understanding of the risks and benefits of vaccines, empowering individuals to make informed decisions about their health.

THE COMPLEXITY OF VACCINE SAFETY

Vaccines are designed to protect against serious illnesses, and their widespread use has led to significant public health successes, such as the eradication of smallpox and the dramatic reduction of polio and measles. However, like any medical intervention, vaccines carry potential risks. While severe side effects are rare, they do occur and can have lasting consequences for those affected.

Adverse Reactions: More Than Just Mild Side Effects

Most vaccines are associated with mild side effects, such as pain at the injection site, fever, or fatigue. These reactions are generally short-lived and considered a normal response as the body builds immunity. However, some individuals experience more severe adverse reactions that go beyond these common symptoms.

Serious side effects, though rare, can include severe allergic reactions (anaphylaxis), seizures, and high fevers. In certain cases, individuals may develop Guillain-Barré syndrome (GBS), a rare neurological disorder characterized by muscle weakness and paralysis. The connection between vaccines and GBS, although uncommon, has been observed with certain vaccines, such as the influenza vaccine. Additionally, reports of myocarditis (inflammation of the heart muscle) following COVID-19 vaccination, particularly among young males, have raised concerns about the long-term effects of certain vaccines.

Autoimmune Reactions and Chronic Health Conditions

There is ongoing debate about the role vaccines may play in triggering autoimmune disorders, where the immune system mistakenly attacks the body's own tissues. Some individuals report developing autoimmune diseases, such as lupus, rheumatoid arthritis, or multiple sclerosis, following vaccination. While the scientific community has not reached a consensus on this issue, the possibility that vaccines could contribute to autoimmune reactions in susceptible individuals cannot be entirely dismissed.

The concern is that certain ingredients in vaccines, such as adjuvants (substances added to enhance the immune response), may stimulate the immune system excessively, leading to unintended effects. Aluminum-based adjuvants, for example, have been linked in some studies to immune dysfunction. Additionally, the use of preservatives like thimerosal, which contains ethylmercury, has been a point of controversy, particularly regarding its potential neurological impact.

Neurological and Developmental Concerns

One of the most contentious issues in the vaccine debate is the potential link between vaccines and neurological conditions, including autism and developmental delays. While numerous studies have found no definitive evidence linking vaccines to autism, many parents continue to express concerns, often citing a temporal relationship between vaccination and the onset of symptoms. It is important to recognize that while the scientific consensus rejects a direct causal link, the lived experiences of families who believe their children were affected by vaccines should not be ignored.

Beyond autism, there are concerns about other potential neurological effects, such as seizures, tics, and attention-deficit/ hyperactivity disorder (ADHD). Some researchers have called for more comprehensive studies to investigate the long-term neurological impact of the increasing number of vaccines given during early childhood. The potential cumulative effects of multiple vaccines, particularly when administered together, are not fully understood, and more research is needed to evaluate the risks for vulnerable populations.

ADDRESSING VACCINE SAFETY CONCERNS

Public health messaging has largely focused on the benefits of vaccines, often dismissing concerns about safety as misinformation or anti-vaccine rhetoric. However, dismissing these concerns outright can create distrust and fuel vaccine hesitancy. Acknowledging the potential risks and addressing them transparently is essential for building public trust and allowing individuals to make informed health decisions.

The Need for Transparent Communication

One of the main issues fueling vaccine hesitancy is the perception that public health authorities and pharmaceutical companies are not forthcoming about the risks associated with vaccines. The push for universal vaccination, while well-intentioned, can sometimes overlook the need for transparency about potential side effects. By providing clear, balanced information that includes both the benefits and risks of vaccination, health authorities can help individuals make more informed choices.

Informed consent is a cornerstone of medical ethics, and patients have the right to know about potential risks before receiving any medical intervention, including vaccines. Public health campaigns should present accurate data on vaccine safety, including statistics on adverse reactions, so that individuals can weigh the risks and benefits based on their personal health history and circumstances.

Strengthening Vaccine Safety Monitoring Systems

To address safety concerns, it is crucial to enhance the systems used to monitor and report adverse vaccine reactions. The Vaccine Adverse Event Reporting System (VAERS) is a valuable tool for tracking potential side effects, but it relies on voluntary reporting, which may lead to underreporting or incomplete data. Strengthening VAERS and similar systems with more rigorous data collection and analysis can help identify potential safety issues more quickly and accurately.

Additionally, conducting long-term studies that follow individuals who have experienced adverse reactions can provide valuable insights into the potential long-term consequences of vaccination. This kind of research can help identify risk factors for severe reactions, allowing for more personalized vaccination recommendations.

INDIVIDUAL SOLUTIONS: INFORMED DECISION-MAKING

When it comes to making decisions about vaccinations, individuals and families should be empowered to take a proactive, informed approach. Here are some steps to consider:

- **Research the Risks and Benefits.** Educate yourself about the potential risks and benefits of each vaccine, using reputable sources such as the Centers for Disease Control and Prevention (CDC) and peer-reviewed medical journals. Understanding the full picture can help you make more informed decisions.
- **Consult Healthcare Providers.** Have open and honest conversations with your healthcare provider about your concerns, especially if you or your child have a history of allergies, autoimmune conditions, or neurological issues. Discuss the possibility of alternative vaccination schedules if you have concerns about the timing or number of vaccines administered.
- **Report Adverse Reactions.** If you or a loved one experience any unusual or severe symptoms following a vaccination, report them to VAERS. This helps contribute to the monitoring of vaccine safety and may aid in identifying potential risks.

GOVERNMENT SOLUTIONS: ENSURING SAFE VACCINATION PRACTICES

The government has a key role in addressing vaccine safety concerns and building public trust. To improve vaccine safety, the following steps should be taken:

- **Enhance Vaccine Safety Research.** Increase funding for independent research on vaccine safety, focusing on potential long-term effects, neurological outcomes, and autoimmune reactions. Prioritizing transparency in this research can help build trust with the public.
- **Improve Informed Consent.** Ensure that healthcare providers offer detailed information about the risks and benefits of vaccines, allowing patients and parents to make truly informed decisions. Standardized, easy-to-understand materials should be provided to explain potential side effects.
- **Personalize Vaccine Recommendations.** Instead of a one-size-fits-all approach, consider implementing more individualized vaccination guidelines that take into account personal health history, genetic predispositions, and known risk factors for adverse reactions.

By taking these steps, public health authorities can address valid safety concerns, provide better guidance, and foster a more balanced understanding of vaccination. Recognizing that vaccines are not without risks, while still emphasizing their role in preventing serious diseases, is key to building a healthier and more informed society.

DR. CRANDALL'S AMERICA:
Combating Health Misinformation

As a doctor, I've seen the devastating impact of health misinformation on my patients, their families, and entire communities. In recent years, misinformation has reached unprecedented levels, fueled by social media and distrust in institutions. This has created a dangerous landscape where patients struggle to discern fact from fiction, often leading to poor health decisions with far-reaching consequences.

One of the most heartbreaking cases I encountered was Sarah, a young mother who came to me with her three-year-old son. Her child was severely underweight and had recurring respiratory infections, which she had been treating with natural remedies she found online. Sarah had avoided vaccinating her son because she feared it would cause autism—something she had read repeatedly on social media. "I just want to protect him," she said tearfully when I explained the risks of her decision. While we worked together to bring her son's health back on track, her story underscored how misinformation can turn even the most well-intentioned parents into victims of false narratives.

Another patient, Tom, refused a potentially life-saving COVID-19 vaccine despite his high-risk status due to chronic heart disease. "I've read too many stories about people getting sick or worse after the shot," he told me. No amount of evidence I provided could convince him otherwise. Tragically, Tom contracted COVID-19 six months later and spent weeks in the ICU. While he survived, his recovery was long and fraught with complications that might have been avoided. His case haunts me because it reflects how misinformation, when unchecked, can have dire, irreversible consequences.

Yet, I've also seen moments of hope—times when misinformation was replaced with understanding through education and compassion. One memorable instance involved a patient named Linda, who was hesitant about receiving the flu vaccine. She admitted, "I've always heard it doesn't really work and can make you sick." Instead of dismissing her concerns, I took the time to explain how the vaccine works, its benefits, and the rare risks. Over time, Linda not only got the flu vaccine but also encouraged her family to do the same. Her transformation reinforced my belief in the power of patient education and open dialogue.

Working in underserved communities has further exposed me to how misinformation thrives where access to reliable information is limited. In one neighborhood, I encountered a group of parents who believed their children didn't need routine vaccinations because "those diseases don't exist anymore." Their lack of awareness stemmed not from willful ignorance but from a lack of access to trustworthy healthcare professionals. It became clear to me that combating misinformation requires more than correcting falsehoods—it requires rebuilding trust in healthcare and making accurate information widely accessible.

I've also witnessed how misinformation impacts providers like myself. Many of my colleagues and I have faced hostility from patients who believe we're part of some grand conspiracy. I remember one patient accusing me of "pushing vaccines for profit," a claim that couldn't be further from the truth. These encounters are deeply frustrating, but they also motivate me to continue advocating for transparency and evidence-based practices.

Despite the challenges, there have been instances of progress. I've worked with schools to implement vaccine education programs, attended community town halls to address fears, and partnered with local leaders to promote health literacy. These efforts don't always yield immediate results, but they plant the seeds of understanding that can grow over time.

What I've learned through these experiences is that combating health misinformation isn't just about providing facts—it's about listening to concerns, building trust, and fostering open conversations. It's about meeting people where they are, without judgment, and helping them navigate the overwhelming sea of information they face daily.

Misinformation is a formidable opponent, but it's not unbeatable. Through persistence, compassion, and education, I've seen how even the most deeply held misconceptions can be overcome. As a doctor, I remain committed to empowering my patients with the knowledge they need to make informed decisions—because their lives, and the health of our communities, depend on it.

R℞ Dr. Crandall's Prescription for Combating Health Misinformation

✔ **Verify Health Information from Reliable Sources.** Cross-check medical claims with reputable sources such as the CDC, WHO, or peer-reviewed research before making health decisions.

✔ **Be Cautious with Social Media Health Advice.** Avoid blindly trusting health information shared on social media without verifying its accuracy, as misinformation spreads quickly online.

✔ **Ask Your Doctor Questions About Treatments and Vaccines.** Engage in open conversations with healthcare providers to clarify risks, benefits, and alternatives before making medical decisions.

✔ **Read Medication and Vaccine Inserts.** Take time to understand the potential side effects and benefits of any prescribed medication or vaccine by reviewing official package inserts and scientific literature.

✔ **Stay Skeptical of "Miracle Cures."** Be wary of products or treatments that claim to cure all diseases, have no side effects, or are marketed as "secret" solutions that mainstream medicine ignores.

✔ **Encourage Critical Thinking in Your Community.** Help friends and family learn how to assess health claims critically, promoting informed discussions rather than fear-based decisions.

✔ **Report and Challenge False Health Claims.** If you encounter misleading medical information online or in your community, report it or respectfully share evidence-based insights to prevent harm.

Resources

National Institutes of Health (NIH)
The U.S. government's comprehensive source for health information, research and clinical updates (https://www.nih.gov).

Centers for Disease Control and Prevention (CDC).
The U.S. national public health institute, providing accurate information on health conditions and diseases (https://www.cdc.gov).

U.S. Department of Health and Human Services
Provides an online toolkit on how to spot health misinformation (https://www.hhs.gov/surgeongeneral/reports-and-publications/health-misinformation/index.html).

How to Report Vaccine Side Effects (VAERS)

A fact sheet about the VAERS system for reporting vaccine side effects, along with the clickable links (https://www.cdc.gov/vaccine -safety-systems/media/pdfs/vaers-factsheet1-p.pdf?CDC_AArefVal =https://www.cdc.gov/vaccinesafety/pdfvaers_factsheet1.pdf).

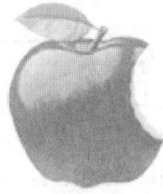

CHAPTER TEN

THE CORPORATE INFLUENCE ON HEALTH

The relationship between corporations and public health is complex and often fraught with tension. On the one hand, businesses are essential to the economy, providing jobs, innovation, and consumer goods that improve the quality of life. On the other hand, the influence of large corporations—particularly those in the food, pharmaceutical, and healthcare industries—has had a profound and often negative impact on public health. Corporate interests can conflict with the goal of improving population health, particularly when profits are prioritized over the well-being of consumers.

From the marketing of unhealthy foods to the lobbying efforts that shape health policy, corporations wield significant power over the health of individuals and communities. This chapter explores the ways in which corporate influence affects public health, the tactics used by corporations to shape health behaviors and policies, and how regulatory frameworks and corporate responsibility can work to mitigate the negative impacts of business interests on health outcomes. It also highlights examples of both harmful corporate practices and initiatives where companies have contributed positively to public health.

HOW CORPORATE INTERESTS
SHAPE PUBLIC HEALTH

Corporate influence on public health is multifaceted, with businesses impacting health both directly, through the products and services they provide, and indirectly, through their lobbying, advertising, and policymaking activities. Large corporations, particularly those in industries related to food, pharmaceuticals, alcohol, and tobacco, have a vested interest in promoting products that may not always align with public health goals. In many cases, the financial success of these industries depends on consumers purchasing products that are harmful to their health, whether it's sugary drinks, fast food, cigarettes, or unnecessary medications.

One of the most visible ways that corporations influence public health is through *marketing and advertising*. Food and beverage companies, for example, spend billions of dollars each year marketing products high in sugar, salt, and fat, particularly to children. Studies have shown that children are especially susceptible to advertising and that exposure to marketing for unhealthy foods can influence their dietary preferences, leading to increased consumption of junk food and sugary drinks. The fast food industry alone spends nearly $5 billion annually on advertising aimed at children and teenagers, contributing to the obesity epidemic in the United States.

The *tobacco industry* provides another clear example of how corporate interests can undermine public health. Despite decades of evidence linking smoking to cancer, heart disease, and other serious health conditions, tobacco companies have continued to market their products aggressively, particularly in low-income and developing countries where regulations are weaker. The industry has also used sophisticated lobbying and public relations campaigns to delay or weaken regulations that could reduce smoking rates. For example, tobacco companies have long fought against plain packaging laws, advertising restrictions, and higher taxes on cigarettes, even though these measures have been shown to reduce smoking rates and improve public health outcomes.

Similarly, the *alcohol industry* has a vested interest in promoting the consumption of its products, even though excessive alcohol use is a leading cause of preventable death and disease. Alcohol companies use targeted marketing campaigns to promote their products, particularly among young adults, often downplaying the risks associated with excessive drinking. At the same time, the industry has worked to influence public policy, lobbying against measures such as alcohol taxes, restrictions on advertising, and limits on sales that could reduce harmful drinking.

In the *pharmaceutical industry*, corporate influence plays out in both the development of new drugs and the marketing of existing ones. While the pharmaceutical industry has made significant contributions to public health by developing life-saving medications and vaccines, it has also been criticized for prioritizing profits over patient well-being. One of the most significant issues is the practice of *direct-to-consumer advertising* (DTCA) of prescription drugs, which is only legal in the United States and New Zealand. DTCA encourages patients to ask their doctors for specific medications, often based on marketing claims rather than medical need. This has led to the overprescription of certain drugs, such as opioids, which has contributed to the opioid crisis in the United States.

In addition to advertising, pharmaceutical companies use *lobbying* and *campaign contributions* to influence health policy. The industry spends billions of dollars each year lobbying Congress and other government bodies to shape regulations and policies in ways that benefit its bottom line. This has led to policies that favor pharmaceutical companies, such as extending patent protections for drugs, delaying the introduction of generic medications, and keeping drug prices high. These practices can limit access to affordable medications, particularly for low-income individuals and those without health insurance.

THE INFLUENCE OF CORPORATE LOBBYING ON HEALTH POLICY

Corporate lobbying is a powerful tool that businesses use to influence health policy in ways that align with their financial interests. Large corporations, particularly those in industries that have a direct impact on public health, such as food, pharmaceuticals, and alcohol, spend vast sums of money each year lobbying lawmakers to shape policies in their favor. While lobbying is a legal and legitimate part of the democratic process, it can sometimes lead to policies that prioritize corporate profits over public health.

One of the most well-documented examples of corporate lobbying's impact on health policy is the *sugar industry's influence* on dietary guidelines and public health research. In the 1960s, the Sugar Research Foundation, an industry group, funded research that downplayed the role of sugar in heart disease and instead shifted the blame to dietary fat. These findings shaped dietary guidelines for decades, leading to a widespread belief that fat, rather than sugar, was the primary culprit in heart disease and obesity. As a result, food companies began producing low-fat, high-sugar products that were marketed as "healthy" alternatives, even though they contributed to the rise in obesity and related health problems.

Corporate lobbying also plays a significant role in shaping *agricultural policies* that impact the food system. For example, large agribusinesses and food corporations have successfully lobbied for subsidies and trade policies that benefit the production of commodity crops like corn, soy, and wheat. These crops are the primary ingredients in many processed foods, and the overproduction of these crops has led to a food system that prioritizes cheap, calorie-dense foods over healthier options like fruits and vegetables. This has contributed to the obesity epidemic and other diet-related health problems in the United States.

The *pharmaceutical industry* is another powerful lobbying force in the United States, spending more on lobbying than any other industry. Pharmaceutical companies lobby for policies that protect their profits, such as patent extensions that delay the introduction of cheaper generic drugs. They also lobby against policies that would lower drug prices, such as allowing Medicare to negotiate drug prices or importing cheaper medications from other countries. These efforts have contributed to the high cost of prescription drugs in the United States, which limits access to life-saving medications for many patients.

Corporate-funded research is another tool that businesses use to influence public health policy. By funding studies that support their products or downplay their risks, corporations can shape the scientific evidence that informs policy decisions. For example, the tobacco industry funded research for decades that downplayed the health risks of smoking, while the alcohol industry has funded studies that emphasize the potential health benefits of moderate drinking. These industry-funded studies can create confusion and undermine public trust in science, making it more difficult for policymakers to implement evidence-based health policies.

CORPORATE SOCIAL RESPONSIBILITY AND PUBLIC HEALTH

While much of the focus on corporate influence in public health is negative, there are also examples of companies taking steps to improve health outcomes through *corporate social responsibility* (CSR) initiatives. CSR refers to the voluntary efforts that businesses make to operate in ways that are ethical, sustainable, and beneficial to society. Many companies, particularly in the food and beverage industry, have implemented CSR initiatives aimed at promoting healthier products, improving access to nutrition, and addressing environmental sustainability.

One notable example of CSR in action is Unilever's Sustainable Living Plan, which includes a commitment to improving the health and well-being of one billion people by 2030. The company has taken steps to reformulate many of its products to reduce sugar, salt, and fat, and it has invested in marketing campaigns that promote healthy eating and physical activity. Unilever has also partnered with public health organizations and governments to address issues like malnutrition and food insecurity in developing countries.

Similarly, Nestlé has implemented a number of CSR initiatives aimed at improving nutrition and public health. The company has committed to reducing sugar, salt, and trans fats in its products and has introduced portion-controlled packaging to encourage healthier eating habits. Nestlé has also invested in nutrition education programs and has worked to improve access to clean water and sanitation in communities where it operates.

In the pharmaceutical industry, some companies have taken steps to improve access to medications for low-income individuals and those in developing countries. For example, Gilead Sciences has implemented a program that provides HIV medications at reduced prices in low- and middle-income countries. Similarly, Novartis has established a global health initiative aimed at addressing non-communicable diseases in low-income populations by providing affordable medications and strengthening healthcare infrastructure.

While CSR initiatives can have a positive impact on public health, there is often skepticism about the motives behind these efforts. Critics argue that CSR programs are often driven by public relations goals rather than a genuine commitment to improving health outcomes. For example, food and beverage companies that promote healthier products or sponsor public health campaigns may still continue to market unhealthy products, particularly in low-income and minority communities. Similarly, pharmaceutical companies that provide access to medications in developing countries may still engage in practices that keep drug prices high in wealthier markets.

HOLDING CORPORATIONS ACCOUNTABLE FOR PUBLIC HEALTH

Given the significant influence that corporations have on public health, it is essential to have mechanisms in place to hold businesses accountable for their impact on health outcomes. This can be achieved through a combination of regulation, consumer advocacy, and corporate responsibility initiatives.

Government regulation is one of the most effective tools for holding corporations accountable for their impact on public health. Regulations that restrict the marketing of unhealthy products, such as tobacco, alcohol, and junk food, can reduce the consumption of these products and improve health outcomes. For example, many countries have implemented bans on tobacco advertising, restrictions on the marketing of sugary drinks to children, and taxes on unhealthy foods. These policies have been shown to reduce consumption and improve public health.

In addition to regulation, *consumer advocacy* plays a critical role in holding corporations accountable for their impact on health. Consumer advocacy groups can raise awareness about the health risks associated with certain products, lobby for stronger regulations, and encourage companies to adopt healthier practices. For example, organizations like the Center for Science in the Public Interest (CSPI) have been instrumental in advocating for nutrition labeling, restrictions on junk food marketing, and reductions in sodium levels in processed foods. These efforts have led to significant changes in food policy and industry practices.

Corporate accountability can also be achieved through *shareholder activism*, where investors use their influence to push companies toward more responsible practices. In recent years, there has been a growing movement of socially responsible investors who prioritize environmental, social, and governance (ESG) factors in their investment decisions. These investors can pressure companies to improve their health and environmental practices by filing shareholder resolutions, engaging in dialogue with corporate management, and voting on key issues at annual meetings.

Finally, *public health partnerships* among governments, non-governmental organizations (NGOs), and the private sector can help ensure that corporations contribute positively to public health. By working together, these stakeholders can develop initiatives that promote healthier products, improve access to nutrition, and address social determinants of health. For example, public-private partnerships have been used to address malnutrition in developing countries, improve access to vaccines, and reduce the environmental impact of food production.

CONCLUSION: BALANCING CORPORATE INTERESTS AND PUBLIC HEALTH

The influence of corporations on public health is both profound and pervasive. While businesses have made significant contributions to economic growth and innovation, their impact on health outcomes is often negative, particularly when profit motives conflict with public health goals. The marketing of unhealthy products, the manipulation of scientific research, and the lobbying efforts to shape health policy in favor of corporate interests have all contributed to rising rates of obesity, chronic disease, and preventable death.

However, there are also opportunities for corporations to play a positive role in improving public health through responsible business practices, corporate social responsibility initiatives, and partnerships with public health organizations. By holding companies accountable for their impact on health and encouraging them to adopt healthier, more sustainable practices, we can create a more balanced relationship between corporate interests and public well-being.

Ultimately, creating a healthier society will require a combination of regulatory frameworks, consumer advocacy, and corporate responsibility. By working together, governments, businesses, and individuals can help ensure that corporate influence aligns with the goal of improving public health outcomes for all.

DR. CRANDALL'S AMERICA:
Battling Corporate Influence on Health

Throughout my career, I've seen how corporate interests shape not only the health choices available to my patients but also their perceptions of what is healthy. The influence of corporations on public health—through food, medication, and healthcare policies—has created a system where profit often takes precedence over well-being. These dynamics have led to some of the most frustrating moments in my practice, but they've also fueled my resolve to advocate for systemic change.

One particularly troubling case involved Linda, a 42-year-old woman battling obesity and prediabetes. Linda struggled to make healthier food choices because her community was inundated with fast food chains and convenience stores. When I asked about her diet, she said, "It's what's cheap and easy, Doc." Linda's struggle wasn't just about personal responsibility—it was a reflection of how the food industry aggressively markets high-calorie, low-nutrient products, especially in low-income areas. The billions spent on advertising junk food far outweigh the resources dedicated to promoting healthy eating, making it harder for patients like Linda to make informed decisions.

I've also seen the impact of pharmaceutical companies on my patients' trust and decision-making. A patient named John came to me with severe side effects from a newly marketed cholesterol medication. He had seen glowing advertisements promising dramatic results but hadn't been told about the potential risks. "Why didn't they tell me this could happen?" he asked. His frustration was justified, as aggressive marketing often downplays risks while overstating benefits, leaving patients like John feeling misled and betrayed.

Another patient, Marsha, was a mother trying to navigate the overwhelming number of "health" products marketed for children. She brought her five-year-old son to me, concerned about his sugar intake after realizing the "healthy" granola bars and fruit snacks she'd been buying were packed with added sugars. "I thought I was doing the right thing," she said. Marsha's case is a stark reminder of how deceptive labeling and marketing can confuse even the most conscientious consumers.

But it's not just food and pharmaceuticals. I've encountered patients who delayed necessary care because they were saddled with high healthcare costs. Many insurance companies prioritize profits over patient access, creating a system where even insured individuals struggle to afford life-saving treatments. One patient, Tom, needed a specific heart medication that wasn't covered by his insurance plan. "I can't afford it, Doc. What's the point of having insurance if it doesn't cover what I need?" he asked. Tom's frustration highlights how corporate practices in the insurance industry often leave patients feeling abandoned by the very system meant to protect them.

Yet, amid these challenges, I've also seen inspiring examples of resistance to corporate influence. In one community, a local coalition successfully campaigned to remove soda machines from schools, replacing them with water stations and healthier snack options. I treated a teenager from that school who said, "It's easier to make good choices now." Small victories like this remind me that change is possible when communities push back against harmful corporate practices.

I've also seen patients like Karen, who was initially hesitant about generic medications after being bombarded with advertisements suggesting they were inferior to brand-name drugs. With education and reassurance, Karen tried the generic option and found it equally effective at a fraction of the cost. "I never realized how much the ads were influencing me," she admitted. Her experience underscores the importance of empowering patients with accurate information to counter misleading corporate messaging.

What these stories have taught me is that corporate influence on health isn't just an abstract problem—it's a daily reality for my patients. From the food they eat to the medications they take, corporate interests shape nearly every aspect of their health journey. While there are moments of progress, the system remains skewed in favor of profit, often at the expense of patient well-being.

As a doctor, I've learned that advocating for my patients means more than treating their conditions—it means helping them navigate a system often designed to exploit their vulnerabilities. By educating patients, supporting community initiatives, and pushing for policy reforms, we can begin to shift the balance of power back to where it belongs: in the hands of those striving to live healthier lives. The fight against corporate influence is far from over, but with persistence and collaboration, I believe we can create a system that prioritizes people over profits.

R℞ Dr. Crandall's Prescription for Safeguarding the Corporate Influence on Health

✔ **Be a Conscious Consumer.** Research the companies behind the food, medications, and healthcare services you use to ensure they prioritize health over profit.

✔ **Read Ingredient Labels Carefully.** Avoid processed foods with harmful additives, preservatives, and excessive sugar, which are often marketed as "healthy" by major corporations.

✔ **Support Ethical and Transparent Brands.** Choose companies that prioritize sustainability, health-conscious ingredients, and ethical business practices over those that focus solely on profit.

✔ **Advocate for Healthier Workplace Policies.** Encourage employers to offer wellness programs, healthier cafeteria options, and better work-life balance to support long-term employee health.

✔ **Be Skeptical of Aggressive Pharmaceutical Marketing.** Understand that direct-to-consumer drug advertisements often highlight benefits while downplaying risks—always consult with a healthcare provider before considering new medications.

✔ **Use Your Purchasing Power for Change.** Support local farmers, independent health stores, and businesses committed to promoting real health solutions rather than corporate-driven convenience.

✔ **Educate Others About Corporate Influence.** Share knowledge with family and friends about how marketing, lobbying, and policy influence public health choices, empowering them to make informed decisions.

Resources

USDA Certified Organic: Understanding the Basics
An informative webpage that explains what the different types of organic labels mean, as well as providing tools and links for both consumers and retailers (https://www.ams.usda.gov/services/organic -certification/organic-basics).

How to Understand and Use the Nutrition Fact Label
How to understand and use the Nutrition Fact Label found on foods (https://www.fda.gov/food/nutrition-facts-label/how-understand -and-use-nutrition-facts-label).

Buying & Using Medicine Safely
A guide to safely buying prescription and over-the-counter drugs (https://www.fda.gov/drugs/information-consumers-and-patients -drugs/buying-using-medicine-safely).

Occupational Safety and Health Administration (OSHA)
A Safe Workplace is Sound Business. Ways to evaluate your workplace safety, with links to resources (https://www.osha.gov/safety -management).

Find Drugs and Conditions
An A-to-Z comprehensive guide to drugs, which includes side effects, a drug interaction checker, and more, tailored for both consumers and professionals (www.drugs.com).

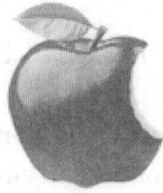

CHAPTER ELEVEN

HEALTH EQUITY: BRIDGING THE GAPS

Health equity is the idea that every person, regardless of race, socioeconomic status, or geographic location, should have an equal opportunity to achieve optimal health. However, in the United States and many other parts of the world, significant disparities in health outcomes exist across different populations. These disparities are driven by a variety of social, economic, and environmental factors, including income inequality, discrimination, lack of access to healthcare, and the social determinants of health.

Health inequities are more than just a public health issue—they are a matter of social justice. The COVID-19 pandemic highlighted these disparities, with marginalized groups, including people of color, low-income individuals, and rural populations, bearing a disproportionate burden of illness and death. Achieving health equity requires addressing both the systemic issues that create disparities and the individual factors that affect health outcomes. This chapter will explore the causes of health disparities, how they manifest in different populations, and the strategies needed to bridge the gaps and ensure health equity for all.

UNDERSTANDING HEALTH DISPARITIES

Health disparities refer to differences in health outcomes that are closely linked to social, economic, and environmental disadvantages. These disparities are often the result of structural inequities, such as racism, poverty, and inadequate healthcare systems, that create barriers to good health for certain populations. In the United States, health disparities are particularly pronounced among racial and ethnic minorities, low-income communities, and rural populations.

One of the most significant factors contributing to health disparities is *race and ethnicity*. In the United States, African Americans, Hispanic/ Latino Americans, Native Americans, and some Asian American subgroups experience higher rates of chronic diseases, such as diabetes, heart disease, and cancer, compared to their white counterparts. For example, African Americans are nearly twice as likely to be diagnosed with diabetes as non-Hispanic whites, and they face a higher risk of complications such as amputations and kidney failure. Similarly, Native Americans have some of the highest rates of obesity, diabetes, and heart disease in the country, largely due to historical and ongoing systemic inequities, including the displacement of Indigenous communities, poor access to healthcare, and food insecurity.

Income inequality also plays a major role in determining health outcomes. Low-income individuals are more likely to experience poor health due to a range of factors, including limited access to nutritious food, safe housing, quality education, and healthcare services. People living in poverty are more likely to suffer from chronic stress, which has been linked to higher rates of heart disease, mental health disorders, and other chronic conditions. In addition, those with lower incomes are less likely to have health insurance or the financial means to pay for necessary medical care, leading to delays in seeking treatment and worse health outcomes.

Geographic disparities also contribute to health inequities. Rural populations often face unique challenges in accessing healthcare due to a lack of healthcare facilities, healthcare providers, and transportation options. Rural areas tend to have higher rates of poverty, lower rates of health insurance coverage, and limited access to specialized care. This can result in poorer health outcomes for conditions such as cancer, heart disease, and stroke. The opioid crisis, for example, has disproportionately affected rural communities, where access to addiction treatment and mental health services is limited.

Education is another social determinant of health that contributes to disparities. Individuals with lower levels of education are more likely to engage in unhealthy behaviors, such as smoking and poor diet, and are less likely to access preventive healthcare services. Education also influences health literacy, or the ability to understand and use health information to make informed decisions. Lower levels of health literacy can lead to poor management of chronic conditions, reduced adherence to medication, and a lack of understanding of preventive measures, such as vaccinations and cancer screenings.

THE INTERSECTION OF HEALTH AND SOCIAL JUSTICE

Health disparities are deeply rooted in broader social justice issues, such as systemic racism, discrimination, and economic inequality. These social determinants of health create unequal opportunities for individuals and communities to achieve good health. For example, racial and ethnic minorities often experience discrimination in healthcare settings, leading to lower-quality care, misdiagnosis, and worse outcomes. A landmark study published in the *Journal of the American Medical Association* (JAMA) found that African American patients are less likely than white patients to receive appropriate care for heart disease, cancer, and diabetes, even after controlling for income and insurance status.

Systemic racism in healthcare is not limited to individual interactions between patients and providers. It is embedded in the policies and practices of healthcare institutions and public health systems. For example, racial segregation in housing has led to the creation of predominantly minority neighborhoods that lack access to healthcare facilities, healthy food options, and safe environments for physical activity. These "health deserts" contribute to higher rates of obesity, diabetes, and other chronic diseases in these communities.

In addition to racism, *gender disparities* affect health outcomes. Women, particularly women of color, often face discrimination in healthcare settings and are less likely to receive adequate care for conditions such as heart disease, which is the leading cause of death among women. Women of color are also at higher risk of maternal mortality and complications during childbirth. In fact, Black women in the United States are three to four times more likely to die from pregnancy-related causes than white women, due in part to systemic racism and unequal access to prenatal care.

LGBTQ+ individuals also face health disparities due to discrimination, stigma, and a lack of culturally competent care. LGBTQ+ individuals are more likely to experience mental health disorders, substance abuse, and barriers to accessing healthcare, particularly for transgender individuals seeking gender-affirming care. These disparities are exacerbated by policies that limit access to healthcare services for LGBTQ+ people, such as insurance exclusions for transgender healthcare.

ADDRESSING THE SOCIAL DETERMINANTS OF HEALTH

Achieving health equity requires addressing the social determinants of health—the conditions in which people are born, grow, live, work, and age. These determinants, such as housing, education, employment, and access to healthcare, have a profound impact on health outcomes. To bridge the gap in health disparities, it is essential to address the root causes of inequality and create environments that support healthy behaviors and access to care.

Housing is one of the most important social determinants of health. Poor housing conditions, such as exposure to mold, lead, and overcrowding, can contribute to respiratory illnesses, mental health problems, and infectious diseases. Lack of affordable housing also forces families to make difficult trade-offs between paying for rent and other essentials like food and healthcare. Housing insecurity is associated with higher rates of chronic diseases, mental health disorders, and delayed medical care. Policies that expand access to affordable housing and improve housing conditions are critical for promoting health equity.

Food security is another key determinant of health. Many low-income and minority communities are classified as food deserts—areas that lack access to affordable, healthy food. Without access to fresh fruits, vegetables, and other nutritious foods, individuals are more likely to rely on processed, unhealthy options that contribute to obesity, diabetes, and heart disease. Efforts to increase access to healthy food, such as expanding farmers' markets, improving food assistance programs like SNAP, and supporting urban agriculture, can help reduce health disparities related to diet and nutrition.

Education and employment opportunities are also essential for promoting health equity. Education provides individuals with the knowledge and skills needed to make informed health decisions, while stable employment offers access to health insurance, income security, and workplace wellness programs. Policies that promote early childhood education, improve public schools, and provide job training and employment opportunities for low-income individuals can have a long-term impact on health outcomes.

Access to healthcare is perhaps the most direct determinant of health equity. Expanding health insurance coverage through programs like Medicaid and the Affordable Care Act (ACA) has helped reduce disparities in access to care, particularly among low-income individuals and people of color. However, gaps in coverage still exist, particularly in states that have not expanded Medicaid. In addition, even individuals with insurance may face barriers to care, such as high deductibles, co-pays, and limited access to specialists. Policies that expand healthcare coverage, reduce out-of-pocket costs, and invest in community health centers can help bridge the gap in healthcare access.

SUCCESSFUL INITIATIVES TO REDUCE HEALTH DISPARITIES

There are numerous examples of successful initiatives that have helped reduce health disparities and promote health equity. These initiatives often involve collaboration among healthcare providers, community organizations, policymakers, and public health agencies to address the specific needs of underserved populations.

One example is the National Diabetes Prevention Program (NDPP), a public-private partnership led by the Centers for Disease Control and Prevention (CDC) that aims to prevent type 2 diabetes in at-risk populations. The NDPP offers lifestyle change programs focused on improving diet, increasing physical activity, and losing weight, which have been shown to reduce the risk of developing diabetes by up to 58%. The program has been particularly effective in reaching low-income and minority populations, who are at higher risk of diabetes.

Community health worker (CHW) programs have also been successful in reducing health disparities. CHWs are trusted members of the communities they serve and are trained to provide health education, support, and advocacy to individuals who face barriers to accessing care. CHWs help bridge the gap between healthcare providers and underserved populations by offering culturally competent care, helping patients navigate the healthcare system, and providing social support. Studies have shown that CHW programs can improve health outcomes for chronic diseases like diabetes and hypertension, particularly in low-income and minority communities.

School-based health centers (SBHCs) are another effective strategy for addressing health disparities. SBHCs provide comprehensive healthcare services, including primary care, mental health services, and dental care, to students in underserved communities. By offering care in schools, SBHCs eliminate barriers to access, such as transportation and cost, and ensure that children receive the care they need to stay healthy and succeed academically. Research has shown that students who use SBHCs are more likely to receive preventive care, such as vaccinations and screenings, and are less likely to visit the emergency room.

In addition to these programs, public health campaigns aimed at reducing tobacco use, promoting vaccination, and encouraging healthy eating have helped reduce health disparities. For example, anti-tobacco campaigns that target low-income and minority communities have contributed to significant declines in smoking rates, particularly among African Americans and Hispanics. Similarly, vaccination campaigns that focus on reaching underserved populations have helped increase immunization rates and reduce the spread of preventable diseases.

POLICY RECOMMENDATIONS TO ENSURE HEALTH EQUITY

To achieve health equity, policymakers must address the systemic factors that contribute to health disparities and implement policies that promote equal access to care and healthy living environments. Some key policy recommendations include:

- **Expanding Access to Healthcare.** Universal healthcare coverage is essential for reducing health disparities. Expanding Medicaid in all states, increasing funding for community health centers, and providing subsidies for low-income individuals to purchase insurance through the ACA marketplace can help ensure that everyone has access to affordable, high-quality care.
- **Addressing Social Determinants of Health.** Policymakers should focus on improving the social and economic conditions

that contribute to health disparities. This includes investing in affordable housing, expanding access to nutritious food, improving public transportation, and increasing funding for education and job training programs.

- **Promoting Culturally Competent Care.** Healthcare providers should receive training on cultural competence and implicit bias to ensure that all patients receive respectful and appropriate care. This can help reduce disparities in treatment and improve patient outcomes for minority populations.
- **Strengthening Public Health Infrastructure.** Public health agencies should be adequately funded to implement programs that address the specific needs of underserved populations. This includes expanding public health campaigns, improving data collection on health disparities, and increasing support for community health worker programs.
- **Reducing Environmental Health Risks.** Policies that address environmental health risks, such as air and water pollution, are essential for promoting health equity. Low-income and minority communities are often disproportionately affected by environmental hazards, so efforts to reduce pollution and improve environmental health should prioritize these populations.

CONCLUSION: A PATH TOWARD HEALTH EQUITY

Health equity is not just a goal for public health professionals—it is a fundamental human right. Everyone, regardless of their background or circumstances, deserves the opportunity to live a healthy life. Achieving health equity requires addressing the social determinants of health, reducing barriers to healthcare access, and ensuring that all individuals have the resources and support they need to make healthy choices.

While significant progress has been made in recent years, much work remains to be done. Bridging the gaps in health disparities will require collaboration among healthcare providers, policymakers, community organizations, and individuals. By working together, we can create a more just and equitable healthcare system that serves all people, regardless of their race, income, or geographic location.

DR. CRANDALL'S AMERICA:
Bridging the Health Equity Gap

Throughout my career, I've witnessed the profound impact of health disparities on individuals and communities. The inequities in access to healthcare, nutritious food, safe housing, and preventive services are not abstract concepts to me—they are the lived realities of many of my patients. These disparities not only undermine the health of individuals but also perpetuate cycles of poor outcomes that ripple across generations.

One patient who left a lasting impression on me was Rosa, a 52-year-old woman who came to my office with uncontrolled diabetes. Rosa lived in a low-income neighborhood and worked two jobs, leaving little time or money for regular doctor visits or healthy meals. "I've been trying, but it's so hard," she told me. Her condition had worsened over the years because she hadn't been able to access consistent care or afford the medication she needed. When I asked about her diet, she explained that her local grocery store carried very few fresh fruits or vegetables, and fast food was often her only option. Rosa's story is a stark reminder of how systemic inequities—like food deserts and economic barriers—directly harm health.

I also think of a young man named Jamal, who avoided seeking care for persistent chest pain because he didn't trust the healthcare system. "I feel like no one really listens to people like me," he told me. Jamal's skepticism stemmed from years of feeling dismissed and marginalized during previous medical visits. When we diagnosed him with an early-stage heart condition that could be managed with proper treatment, he was relieved but still hesitant about follow-up care. His case reinforced for me how essential it is to rebuild trust between underserved communities and the medical system.

Another patient, Maria, struggled with mental health issues exacerbated by her circumstances. She was a single mother living in an overcrowded apartment, constantly worried about making ends meet. When I referred her to a mental health counselor, she couldn't find an available provider who accepted her insurance. "It feels like there's no help for people like me," she said. Her situation highlighted the gaps in mental health services, particularly for those in underprivileged communities.

Despite these challenges, I've also seen moments of progress. I worked with a community clinic in a rural area where mobile health units brought care directly to patients who otherwise wouldn't have access to transportation or nearby providers. I'll never forget meeting an elderly woman who had avoided seeking care for years but finally received a diagnosis and treatment for her condition because the clinic came to her. "I didn't think anyone cared," she said. These experiences remind me of the power of innovative solutions in reducing disparities.

One of the most inspiring examples of bridging the health equity gap came from a grassroots initiative I encountered in an inner-city neighborhood. Local leaders partnered with health professionals to establish a farmers' market that accepted food stamps and provided free health screenings. I saw firsthand how this initiative improved not only physical health but also the community's sense of pride and connection. "We're finally being seen," one participant told me. Moments like these remind me that change is possible when communities and healthcare providers work together.

Yet, the systemic challenges remain daunting. I've treated patients who couldn't afford life-saving medications despite having insurance, children who fell behind on vaccinations because their parents couldn't take time off work, and families who faced eviction because of medical bills. These stories underscore how deeply intertwined health is with broader social and economic factors.

What these experiences have taught me is that addressing health equity requires more than treating individual patients—it demands systemic change. Policies that expand access to affordable care, improve housing and transportation, and eliminate food deserts are critical. But equally important are fostering trust, listening to the needs of underserved communities, and tailoring solutions to their specific challenges.

As a doctor, I've seen both the heartbreaking consequences of inequity and the incredible potential for resilience when people are given the resources and respect they deserve. Bridging the health equity gap is one of the most pressing challenges of our time, but it is also one of the most rewarding. Each patient like Rosa, Jamal, or Maria reinforces my commitment to advocating for a system that works for everyone, not just the privileged few. By addressing these disparities head-on, we can create a future where health is not a luxury but a fundamental right for all.

R℞ Dr. Crandall's Prescription for Ensuring Health Equity

✔ **Advocate for Equal Access to Healthcare.** Support policies and initiatives that work to make quality healthcare affordable and accessible to all, regardless of income or location.

✔ **Be Mindful of Social Determinants of Health.** Recognize that factors such as education, income, housing, and transportation play crucial roles in overall well-being, and advocate for solutions that address these disparities.

✔ **Support Community Health Programs.** Engage with, or donate to, local organizations that provide healthcare, nutrition assistance, or wellness programs to underserved populations.

✔ **Encourage Health Literacy in Vulnerable Communities.** Help spread awareness about preventive care, chronic disease management, and healthy lifestyle choices to those who may lack access to proper health education.

✔ **Mentor and Uplift Future Health Advocates.** If you have knowledge or resources, consider mentoring young individuals from disadvantaged backgrounds who aspire to enter the medical or wellness fields.

✔ **Promote Inclusivity in Wellness Spaces.** Encourage the creation of fitness centers, farmers' markets, and health programs that accommodate diverse communities, including people of all income levels and abilities.

✔ **Challenge Discrimination in Healthcare Settings.** Speak up when you witness racial, socioeconomic, or gender-based biases in healthcare, and support efforts to ensure fair treatment for all patients.

Resources

211 Helpline
Dial "211" or visit the website for confidential help on meeting basic needs like housing, food, transportation, and healthcare. This is an excellent resource to pass along to those in need (https://www.211.org).

Families USA
A nonprofit, nonpartisan consumer health advocacy and policy organization working to expand healthcare services (https://www .familiesusa.org).

Patient Advocate Foundation
A national nonprofit organization providing professional case management services to those with chronic, life threatening, and debilitating illness (https://www.patientadvocate.org).

National Council on Interpreting in Health Care
A national organization for people who want to become trained interpreters for patients in healthcare settings (https://www.ncihc.org).

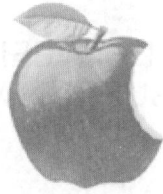

CHAPTER TWELVE

A SUSTAINABLE FUTURE FOR HEALTH

The connection between environmental sustainability and public health is undeniable. The health of our planet directly impacts the health of its inhabitants, from the air we breathe and the water we drink to the food we eat. As climate change accelerates and environmental degradation worsens, the consequences for human health are becoming increasingly apparent. Rising temperatures, extreme weather events, pollution, and the loss of biodiversity are all contributing to a growing global health crisis. In this context, a sustainable future for health is not only desirable—it is essential.

This chapter will explore the intersection of environmental sustainability and public health, examining how environmental factors affect human health and what can be done to mitigate these impacts. It will also discuss the role of healthcare systems in reducing their environmental footprint and how adopting sustainable practices can improve health outcomes. Finally, the chapter will highlight successful initiatives and policies that are paving the way toward a more sustainable future for health.

THE CONNECTION BETWEEN ENVIRONMENTAL SUSTAINABILITY AND PUBLIC HEALTH

The environment plays a critical role in shaping public health outcomes. Clean air, safe drinking water, fertile soils, and stable ecosystems are all essential to human survival and well-being. However, environmental degradation—driven by factors such as pollution, deforestation, industrial agriculture, and fossil fuel consumption—has created significant public health challenges.

One of the most pressing issues is *air pollution*, which is responsible for millions of premature deaths worldwide each year. Fine particulate matter (PM2.5) from vehicle emissions, industrial activities, and power plants can penetrate deep into the lungs, leading to respiratory diseases such as asthma, chronic obstructive pulmonary disease (COPD), and lung cancer. Air pollution also exacerbates cardiovascular diseases, increasing the risk of heart attacks and strokes. Children, the elderly, and individuals with pre-existing health conditions are particularly vulnerable to the effects of poor air quality.

Water pollution is another critical public health issue. Contaminants such as heavy metals, industrial chemicals, and agricultural runoff can contaminate drinking water supplies, leading to a range of health problems, including gastrointestinal diseases, developmental disorders, and even cancer. In some parts of the world, lack of access to clean water is a leading cause of preventable death, particularly among children. Waterborne diseases such as cholera, dysentery, and typhoid fever remain significant public health challenges in regions with inadequate water and sanitation infrastructure.

Climate change is amplifying many of these environmental threats and creating new health risks. Rising global temperatures are contributing to more frequent and severe heatwaves, which can cause heat-related illnesses and deaths, particularly among vulnerable populations such as the elderly and outdoor workers. Climate change is also altering the patterns of infectious diseases, as warming temperatures and shifting ecosystems allow disease-carrying vectors like mosquitoes to expand into new regions. For example, diseases such as malaria, dengue fever, and Lyme disease are becoming more prevalent in areas where they were previously rare.

In addition to direct health impacts, climate change is contributing to *food insecurity* by disrupting agricultural production. Extreme weather events such as droughts, floods, and hurricanes can destroy crops, reduce food yields, and drive up food prices, leading to malnutrition and hunger. These challenges are particularly acute in developing countries, where food systems are more vulnerable to environmental shocks. However, even in wealthier nations, climate change is expected to strain food production and supply chains, potentially leading to shortages of certain foods and higher prices for consumers.

Biodiversity loss is another environmental issue with profound implications for public health. Healthy ecosystems provide a range of services that support human health, including water purification, air filtration, and pollination of crops. Biodiversity also plays a crucial role in regulating disease by maintaining ecological balances that prevent the spread of pathogens. The destruction of natural habitats, deforestation, and the illegal wildlife trade are increasing human exposure to zoonotic diseases—those that can be transmitted from animals to humans. The COVID-19 pandemic, believed to have originated from a wildlife market, is a stark reminder of the links between environmental degradation and global health threats.

SUSTAINABLE HEALTHCARE: REDUCING THE ENVIRONMENTAL FOOTPRINT

The healthcare sector, while dedicated to improving health, is also a significant contributor to environmental degradation. Hospitals, clinics, and healthcare facilities consume large amounts of energy, generate substantial waste, and rely heavily on resource-intensive materials such as plastics, pharmaceuticals, and medical equipment. The carbon footprint of the healthcare sector is substantial, with the World Health Organization (WHO) estimating that healthcare is responsible for approximately 5% of global greenhouse gas emissions.

However, healthcare systems also have a unique opportunity to lead the way in promoting sustainability and reducing their environmental impact. By adopting sustainable practices, healthcare facilities can not only reduce their carbon footprint but also improve health outcomes by creating healthier environments for patients, staff, and surrounding communities.

One of the key strategies for reducing the environmental impact of healthcare is *energy efficiency*. Hospitals are among the most energy-intensive buildings, with large heating, ventilation, and air conditioning (HVAC) systems running around the clock. Transitioning to renewable energy sources such as solar or wind power can significantly reduce a facility's carbon footprint. In addition, energy-efficient lighting, HVAC systems, and building materials can lower energy consumption and reduce operating costs. For example, Kaiser Permanente, one of the largest healthcare providers in the United States, has made a commitment to carbon neutrality and has invested in renewable energy to power its hospitals and clinics.

Waste reduction is another critical area for sustainable healthcare. The healthcare sector generates a vast amount of waste, including single-use plastics, medical supplies, and hazardous materials. While some of this waste is necessary for infection control and patient safety, there are many opportunities to reduce waste through recycling, reusing medical equipment, and minimizing unnecessary packaging. For example, some hospitals have implemented programs to recycle operating room waste, such as unused surgical supplies, and donate them to medical facilities in developing countries.

Sustainable procurement is another key strategy for reducing the healthcare sector's environmental footprint. By choosing environmentally friendly products and suppliers, healthcare organizations can promote sustainability throughout the supply chain. This includes selecting energy-efficient medical equipment, sourcing biodegradable or recyclable materials, and purchasing pharmaceuticals and chemicals from manufacturers that prioritize sustainability. Hospitals can also work with suppliers to reduce the environmental impact of transportation by sourcing goods locally or using lower-emission delivery methods.

In addition to these strategies, healthcare systems can play a leadership role in promoting *environmental health* by advocating for policies that address the root causes of environmental degradation. For example, hospitals and healthcare providers can support clean air and water initiatives, promote policies that reduce carbon emissions, and raise awareness about the health impacts of climate change. By taking a proactive approach to environmental health, healthcare systems can not only improve their own sustainability but also help create healthier communities.

THE CO-BENEFITS OF SUSTAINABILITY FOR HEALTH

One of the key benefits of adopting sustainable practices in healthcare and other sectors is the concept of *co-benefits*—the idea that actions taken to protect the environment can also directly improve human health. Many of the strategies for reducing environmental impact, such as improving air quality, promoting active transportation, and transitioning to renewable energy, have immediate and tangible health benefits for individuals and communities.

For example, *improving air quality* by reducing emissions from vehicles, power plants, and industrial sources can lead to significant reductions in respiratory diseases, heart disease, and premature deaths. A study by the American Lung Association found that transitioning to cleaner energy sources and reducing emissions from transportation could prevent tens of thousands of premature deaths and reduce healthcare costs by billions of dollars each year in the United States alone.

Active transportation—such as walking, cycling, and public transit—offers another important co-benefit. Cities that invest in pedestrian-friendly infrastructure and public transit not only reduce their carbon footprint but also encourage physical activity, which is linked to lower rates of obesity, diabetes, and cardiovascular disease. Active transportation also reduces the risk of traffic-related injuries and improves mental health by reducing stress and increasing social connections.

In the *food system*, adopting sustainable agricultural practices, such as organic farming, regenerative agriculture, and reducing meat consumption, can improve both environmental and public health outcomes. Sustainable farming methods that avoid the use of synthetic pesticides and fertilizers reduce water and soil pollution while also producing healthier food with fewer chemical residues. Reducing the consumption of red and processed meats, which are linked to higher rates of cancer and heart disease, can lower the environmental impact of agriculture and improve population health.

POLICY SOLUTIONS FOR A SUSTAINABLE FUTURE FOR HEALTH

Achieving a sustainable future for health requires coordinated action at the local, national, and global levels. Governments, businesses, healthcare providers, and individuals all have a role to play in reducing environmental degradation and promoting sustainability. Several policy solutions can help drive progress toward a more sustainable and healthier future.

- **Implementing strong environmental regulations.** Governments have a critical role in setting and enforcing environmental standards that protect public health. Policies that limit emissions of greenhouse gases, reduce air and water pollution, and promote the use of renewable energy are essential for mitigating the health impacts of climate change and environmental degradation. For example, the Clean Air Act in the United States has been highly effective in reducing air pollution and improving respiratory health. Expanding and strengthening such regulations is crucial for protecting both the environment and public health.

- **Investing in green infrastructure.** Green infrastructure, such as parks, green roofs, and urban forests, provides multiple environmental and health benefits. Green spaces improve air and water quality, reduce the urban heat island effect, and provide opportunities for physical activity and recreation. Governments and city planners should prioritize the development of green infrastructure in urban areas, particularly in low-income communities that often have limited access to parks and green spaces.

- **Supporting sustainable agriculture.** Agricultural policies should prioritize sustainable farming practices that protect soil health, reduce water use, and minimize the use of harmful chemicals. Governments can incentivize organic and regenerative farming through subsidies, grants, and research funding. In addition, policies that promote plant-based diets and reduce the consumption of resource-intensive foods like red meat can improve both environmental sustainability and public health.

- **Promoting sustainable healthcare systems.** Healthcare systems should be encouraged to adopt sustainable practices, such as energy efficiency, waste reduction, and sustainable procurement. Governments can support these efforts by providing financial incentives for hospitals and clinics to invest in renewable energy and energy-efficient technologies. In addition, healthcare providers can be trained in environmental health and sustainability, enabling them to advocate for policies that protect both the environment and public health.

- **Raising public awareness.** Public health campaigns can play a key role in educating individuals about the connections between environmental sustainability and health. By raising awareness about the health impacts of climate change, air pollution, and food choices, governments and non-governmental organizations (NGOs) can empower individuals to make more sustainable choices in their daily lives. For example, campaigns that promote active transportation, energy conservation, and plant-based diets can help reduce environmental impact while improving health outcomes.

Examples of Successful Initiatives

Several successful initiatives around the world demonstrate the potential for creating a more sustainable future for health.

The Lancet Countdown on Health and Climate Change is a global initiative that tracks the health impacts of climate change and the progress being made to address them. The Lancet Countdown brings together researchers, policymakers, and healthcare providers to promote evidence-based policies that protect both the environment and public health. The initiative has highlighted the co-benefits of climate action for health and has called for urgent action to reduce greenhouse gas emissions and build climate-resilient health systems.

The Health Care Without Harm (HCWH) network is another example of a successful initiative promoting sustainability in healthcare. HCWH works with hospitals and healthcare providers around the world to reduce their environmental footprint through energy efficiency, waste reduction, and sustainable procurement. The network has helped healthcare facilities transition to renewable energy, reduce the use of harmful chemicals, and implement green building practices. By promoting sustainability in healthcare, HCWH is helping to protect both the environment and the health of patients and staff.

In the food sector, the EAT-Lancet Commission on Food, Planet, Health has developed a global framework for healthy and sustainable diets. The Commission's recommendations include reducing the consumption of red and processed meats, increasing the intake of fruits, vegetables, and plant-based proteins, and adopting sustainable farming practices. These changes not only reduce the environmental impact of food production but also improve public health by reducing the risk of chronic diseases such as heart disease, diabetes, and cancer.

CONCLUSION: A SUSTAINABLE FUTURE FOR HEALTH

The health of the planet and the health of its people are inextricably linked. Environmental degradation and climate change are contributing to a growing public health crisis, with rising rates of respiratory diseases, infectious diseases, and food insecurity. However, by adopting sustainable practices and policies, we can mitigate these impacts and create a healthier future for all.

Sustainable healthcare systems, green infrastructure, and sustainable agriculture are key components of a holistic approach to health and sustainability. By reducing the environmental footprint of healthcare, promoting active transportation, and supporting sustainable food systems, we can improve health outcomes while protecting the planet.

Achieving a sustainable future for health will require collaboration among governments, businesses, healthcare providers, and individuals. Together, we can create a world where both the environment and public health thrive, ensuring a better quality of life for current and future generations.

DR. CRANDALL'S AMERICA:
The Connection Between Health and Sustainability

Throughout my career, I've seen the deep interconnection between environmental factors and health. From air and water quality to the sustainability of our food systems, the state of our environment directly impacts the well-being of individuals and communities. Unfortunately, I've also witnessed how environmental neglect and unsustainable practices disproportionately harm vulnerable populations, creating a cycle of illness that is difficult to break.

One patient who stands out is Carla, a 45-year-old mother of three living in an industrial area. She came to me with persistent respiratory problems, and as we delved into her history, it became clear that her health issues were tied to the poor air quality in her neighborhood. Carla lived near a factory that emitted significant pollutants, and she explained how her children often suffered from asthma attacks. "We don't have the option to move," she told me, a heartbreaking reality for so many families like hers. Her story reinforced the link between environmental hazards and chronic health conditions, a connection I've seen repeatedly throughout my career.

Another patient, Greg, a farmer in his sixties, struggled with the long-term effects of pesticide exposure. Over years of conventional farming, Greg had developed neurological symptoms and a weakened immune system. He confided in me, "I always thought I was doing what I needed to feed my family and the community, but I didn't realize it was costing me my health." Greg's case highlights the dangers of unsustainable agricultural practices—not just for the environment, but for the individuals working within these systems.

I've also treated patients affected by the increasing severity of climate-related disasters. One family I worked with had been displaced by a hurricane, losing their home and access to fresh food and clean water. They came to me suffering from malnutrition, dehydration, and stress-related illnesses. "We've lost everything," the mother told me. These experiences have shown me how climate change compounds existing health disparities, leaving the most vulnerable to bear the brunt of its impacts.

Despite these challenges, I've seen moments of progress and hope. In one rural community, I partnered with a group of farmers transitioning to regenerative agriculture. By eliminating harmful pesticides and focusing on soil health, they not only improved their yields but also reduced their exposure to toxins. One farmer told me, "I feel better than I have in years, and I know we're leaving the land in better shape for the next generation." Initiatives like this demonstrate the powerful health benefits of sustainable practices.

In urban areas, I've worked with programs that transformed vacant lots into community gardens. These gardens not only provide fresh, nutritious food but also offer residents a chance to connect with nature and reduce stress. I'll never forget one patient, a woman named Linda, who started gardening after her doctor recommended it for her anxiety. "It's not just about the food," she told me. "It's about feeling alive again." Stories like hers remind me that sustainability isn't just about preserving the planet— it's about creating healthier, more vibrant communities.

However, systemic barriers persist. I've encountered patients who can't afford organic or sustainably produced food, despite knowing it would benefit their health. I've also seen the frustration of community leaders trying to implement green initiatives, only to face resistance from corporations or local governments. These challenges underscore the need for broader policy changes to support environmental sustainability and public health.

What these experiences have taught me is that health and sustainability are inseparable. Clean air, safe water, nutritious food, and a stable climate are foundational to well-being. Yet, achieving these goals requires a collective effort—one that involves policymakers, businesses, healthcare providers, and individuals.

As a doctor, I can treat the symptoms caused by environmental neglect, but real change requires addressing the root causes. By advocating for sustainable practices and policies, I hope to create a future where patients like Carla, Greg, and Linda can thrive in a healthier, more sustainable world. Their stories inspire me to keep pushing for change, because the health of our planet and the health of our people are one and the same.

R℞ Dr. Crandall's Prescription for a Sustainable Future for Health

- ✔ **Reduce Exposure to Environmental Toxins.** Be mindful of air and water quality, and choose organic or chemical-free products when possible to minimize exposure to harmful pollutants.
- ✔ **Support Sustainable and Regenerative Agriculture.** Purchase food from farmers' markets or suppliers who prioritize soil health, biodiversity, and eco-friendly farming practices.
- ✔ **Limit Plastic Use in Food Storage and Packaging.** Reduce reliance on plastic containers, and opt for glass, stainless steel, or other sustainable alternatives to decrease exposure to microplastics and endocrine-disrupting chemicals.

- ✔ **Incorporate More Plant-Based Foods.** Even small changes, such as one meat-free meal per week, can reduce the environmental impact of food production and improve personal health.
- ✔ **Choose Eco-Friendly Personal and Household Products.** Opt for natural, biodegradable cleaning supplies and skincare and hygiene products that don't contribute to pollution or disrupt hormones.
- ✔ **Reduce Food Waste.** Plan meals, store food properly, and compost scraps to minimize waste and promote sustainable consumption habits.
- ✔ **Advocate for Green Spaces in Communities.** Support local efforts to expand parks, urban gardens, and tree-lined streets, which improve air quality, mental health, and overall well-being.

Resources

Safer Choice Program
Information on choosing good, effective products that are safer for the environment (https://www.epa.gov/saferchoice).

What You Can Do to Reduce Plastic Waste
How to reduce plastic waste; includes information on extending the use of plastic products, purchasing used items or donating them for reuse (https://www.epa.gov/plastics/what-you-can-do-reduce -plastic-waste).

Outdoor and Indoor Air Adaptation Strategy for Climate Change
How to reduce air pollution; includes transportation, household and lawn and garden tips (https://www.epa.gov/arc-x/outdoor-and -indoor-air-adaptation-strategies-climate-change).

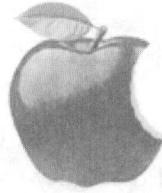

CHAPTER THIRTEEN

MENTAL HEALTH IN THE MODERN WORLD

Mental health is increasingly recognized as a critical component of overall well-being, yet it remains one of the most under-discussed and under-addressed aspects of public health. In the modern world, rapid technological changes, shifting societal norms, and increasing pressures from work and daily life have contributed to a rising tide of mental health challenges. Anxiety, depression, stress, and burnout are more prevalent than ever, affecting people across all age groups and walks of life.

Despite growing awareness, the stigma surrounding mental health persists, and access to mental health services remains a significant barrier for many individuals. This chapter explores the state of mental health in the modern world, the factors contributing to the mental health crisis, and the ways society can better support mental well-being. We will also examine the role of technology in both exacerbating and addressing mental health challenges, and discuss the importance of integrating mental healthcare into broader health and social systems.

THE RISING TIDE OF MENTAL HEALTH ISSUES

In the last few decades, mental health disorders have emerged as one of the leading causes of disability worldwide. According to the World Health Organization (WHO), depression is now the leading cause of disability, affecting more than 264 million people globally. Anxiety disorders, including generalized anxiety disorder (GAD), panic disorder, and social anxiety disorder, affect an estimated 284 million people. Other mental health conditions, such as bipolar disorder, schizophrenia, and post-traumatic stress disorder (PTSD), also contribute significantly to the global burden of disease.

In the United States, the statistics are equally alarming. The National Alliance on Mental Illness (NAMI) reports that one in five adults—about 51.5 million people—experience mental illness each year. Among youth, the numbers are even more concerning, with suicide now the second leading cause of death among individuals aged 10 to 34. The COVID-19 pandemic has only exacerbated these trends, as social isolation, economic hardship, and the uncertainty of the global crisis have led to increased rates of anxiety, depression, and stress.

While the prevalence of mental health issues is growing, awareness and acceptance of mental health disorders have also increased, leading more people to seek help. However, stigma remains a major barrier to treatment. Many individuals feel ashamed or embarrassed to admit they are struggling with their mental health, fearing judgment or misunderstanding from others. This stigma can prevent people from seeking the help they need, leading to worsening symptoms and, in some cases, tragic outcomes such as suicide.

THE CAUSES OF THE MENTAL HEALTH CRISIS

The mental health crisis is the result of a complex interplay of factors, including social, economic, environmental, and biological influences. While each individual's experience with mental health is unique, several broader trends in modern society contribute to the rising rates of mental health disorders.

Economic Pressure and Job Insecurity

One of the most significant contributors to mental health issues in the modern world is the increasing pressure to succeed in a highly competitive economic environment. Globalization, automation, and the rise of the gig economy have created job insecurity for millions of workers, leading to chronic stress and anxiety. People are often forced to work long hours, take on multiple jobs, or accept precarious employment without benefits or job security, all of which can take a toll on mental health.

In addition, the high cost of living, particularly in urban areas, can lead to financial stress, which is closely linked to depression and anxiety. Many individuals struggle to make ends meet, juggling rent, student loans, healthcare costs, and other financial obligations. The stress of trying to stay financially afloat can lead to burnout, a condition characterized by emotional exhaustion, detachment, and decreased productivity, which has become increasingly common in today's workforce.

Social Isolation and Loneliness

While technology has made it easier to stay connected, it has also contributed to a growing sense of social isolation and loneliness, particularly among younger generations. The rise of social media, for example, has changed the way people interact with one another, leading to more superficial connections and fewer meaningful face-to-face interactions. Research has shown that excessive use of social media can contribute to feelings of loneliness, depression, and anxiety, as individuals compare themselves to others and feel inadequate or left out.

In addition to the impact of technology, societal changes such as increased urbanization and the breakdown of traditional social structures have contributed to a sense of disconnection. Many people live far from family and friends, and the support networks that once provided a sense of belonging and security have weakened. The COVID-19 pandemic has further exacerbated social isolation, as lockdowns and social distancing measures have limited opportunities for in-person interactions.

The Pace of Modern Life

The fast pace of modern life, coupled with the pressure to constantly "perform" and be productive, has created a culture of stress and burnout. Many individuals feel overwhelmed by the demands of work, family, and personal life, leading to chronic stress that can take a serious toll on mental health. This constant pressure to succeed and "hustle" is particularly evident in Western cultures, where success is often measured by professional achievements, financial wealth, and material possessions.

In addition to work-related stress, the 24/7 news cycle and the constant barrage of information from social media, email, and smartphones have made it difficult for people to disconnect and relax. The inability to unplug and take breaks can lead to heightened levels of anxiety and feelings of being overwhelmed.

Trauma and Adversity

Experiences of trauma and adversity are significant risk factors for the development of mental health disorders. Childhood trauma, including physical, emotional, or sexual abuse, neglect, and household dysfunction, is strongly linked to mental health problems later in life, including depression, anxiety, PTSD, and substance abuse. In fact, research has shown that individuals who experience multiple adverse childhood experiences (ACEs) are more likely to develop chronic mental health conditions.

Adults who experience trauma, such as violence, natural disasters, accidents, or the loss of a loved one, are also at risk for developing mental health disorders. The cumulative effects of trauma can lead to lasting emotional and psychological scars, affecting a person's ability to cope with stress and maintain healthy relationships.

Biological and Genetic Factors

While environmental and social factors play significant roles in mental health, biological and genetic factors also contribute to an individual's vulnerability to mental health disorders. Research has shown that mental health conditions such as depression, bipolar disorder, schizophrenia, and anxiety disorders have a genetic component, meaning that individuals with a family history of these conditions are more likely to experience them.

In addition, neurochemical imbalances, such as low levels of serotonin or dopamine, can affect mood and behavior. Hormonal changes, particularly during periods such as adolescence, pregnancy, and menopause, can also influence mental health. Understanding the biological underpinnings of mental health disorders is essential for developing effective treatments, but it is important to recognize that mental health is shaped by a complex interplay of biological, psychological, and social factors.

THE ROLE OF TECHNOLOGY IN MENTAL HEALTH

Technology has both exacerbated and helped to address mental health challenges in the modern world. On the one hand, the rise of social media, smartphones, and constant connectivity has contributed to feelings of anxiety, stress, and social isolation. On the other hand, technology has also created new opportunities for improving access to mental health care and providing support to individuals in need.

The Impact of Social Media

Social media platforms such as Facebook, Instagram, and X have become integral to modern life, offering a way for people to stay connected and share their lives with others. However, research has shown that excessive use of social media can have negative effects on mental health, particularly among young people. Studies have found that individuals who spend more time on social media are more likely to experience symptoms of depression, anxiety, and loneliness.

One of the reasons social media can be harmful to mental health is the tendency for individuals to compare themselves to others. On social media, people often present an idealized version of their lives, showcasing their achievements, experiences, and physical appearance. This can create unrealistic expectations and lead to feelings of inadequacy or low self-esteem. In addition, cyberbullying and online harassment are significant issues on social media platforms, particularly for young people, and can contribute to mental health problems such as anxiety, depression, and suicidal thoughts.

Digital Health Tools and Teletherapy

While technology can contribute to mental health challenges, it also offers new solutions for improving mental well-being. One of the most significant advancements in recent years has been the rise of digital mental health tools and teletherapy platforms. These tools provide individuals with convenient, accessible, and affordable ways to manage their mental health and receive professional support.

Teletherapy, or online therapy, allows individuals to connect with licensed mental health professionals from the comfort of their own homes, using video calls, messaging, or phone calls. This was particularly beneficial during the COVID-19 pandemic, when many people were unable or unwilling to attend in-person therapy sessions. Teletherapy has made mental health care more accessible for individuals in rural areas, people with mobility issues, and those who face stigma around seeking help. Studies have shown that teletherapy can be just as effective as in-person therapy for many mental health conditions, including depression and anxiety.

In addition to teletherapy, *mental health apps* have become increasingly popular. These apps offer a range of services, from guided meditation and mindfulness exercises to mood tracking and cognitive-behavioral therapy (CBT) tools. For example, apps like Headspace and Calm provide users with meditation exercises to reduce stress and improve mental well-being, while apps like Moodfit and Youper offer tools for tracking mood and managing anxiety or depression. These digital tools can be particularly helpful for individuals who are not ready to seek professional help but want to take steps to improve their mental health.

Artificial Intelligence and Mental Health

Artificial intelligence (AI) is also playing an emerging role in the field of mental health. AI-powered tools are being developed to help identify individuals at risk for mental health conditions and to provide personalized treatment recommendations. For example, AI algorithms can analyze patterns in a person's speech, writing, or behavior to detect early signs of depression or anxiety. These tools can help mental health professionals make more accurate diagnoses and provide tailored interventions.

AI is also being used to create *virtual therapists*, which can offer support to individuals in real-time. For example, Woebot is an AI-powered chatbot that provides users with cognitive-behavioral therapy exercises and emotional support. While virtual therapists are not a replacement for human mental health professionals, they can provide immediate assistance and serve as a complement to traditional therapy.

ADDRESSING THE MENTAL HEALTH CRISIS

Addressing the mental health crisis in the modern world requires a comprehensive approach that includes improving access to mental healthcare, reducing stigma, and promoting mental well-being at the individual, community, and societal levels.

Expanding Access to Mental Healthcare

One of the most significant barriers to addressing the mental health crisis is the lack of access to affordable and timely mental healthcare. In many parts of the world, mental health services are underfunded, and individuals may face long wait times or high costs for treatment. Even in countries with more robust mental health systems, there are often significant disparities in access to care based on factors such as income, geographic location, and race.

Expanding access to mental health care requires increased investment in mental health services, particularly in underserved communities. This includes training more mental health professionals, integrating mental health care into primary care settings, and providing financial support for individuals who cannot afford treatment. Teletherapy and digital mental health tools can also play a key role in expanding access to care, particularly for individuals who face barriers to in-person services.

Reducing Stigma

Reducing the stigma surrounding mental health is essential for encouraging more people to seek help and for creating a more supportive environment for individuals with mental health conditions. Public awareness campaigns, mental health education in schools, and open conversations about mental health can help challenge stereotypes and misconceptions.

In addition to reducing stigma in society at large, it is important to address the stigma that exists within healthcare settings. Many individuals with mental health conditions report experiencing discrimination or dismissal from healthcare providers, which can discourage them from seeking care. Training healthcare professionals to provide compassionate and culturally competent care is essential for improving mental health outcomes.

Promoting Mental Well-Being

Preventing mental health disorders and promoting mental well-being is just as important as treating mental illness. This requires creating environments that support emotional resilience, reduce stress, and foster healthy relationships. Workplaces, schools, and communities all have roles to play in promoting mental well-being.

Workplaces can implement policies that promote work-life balance, reduce job stress, and provide mental health support to employees. Offering flexible work arrangements, mental health days, and access to counseling services can help prevent burnout and improve employee well-being.

Schools can promote mental well-being by providing mental health education, creating supportive environments for students, and offering resources such as counseling and peer support programs. Teaching children and adolescents about emotional regulation, stress management, and resilience can help them develop the skills they need to navigate life's challenges.

Communities can also play a role in promoting mental well-being by creating spaces for social connection and support. Programs that encourage community building, such as social clubs, volunteer opportunities, and support groups, can help reduce social isolation and foster a sense of belonging.

CONCLUSION: A PATH FORWARD FOR MENTAL HEALTH

Mental health is a critical component of overall well-being, yet it remains a significant challenge in the modern world. Economic pressures, social isolation, the fast pace of life, and trauma all contribute to the rising rates of mental health disorders. Addressing this crisis requires a multi-faceted approach that includes expanding access to mental health care, reducing stigma, and promoting mental well-being at all levels of society.

While technology has contributed to some of the challenges of modern life, it also offers new opportunities for improving mental health. Teletherapy, mental health apps, and AI-powered tools can help make mental health care more accessible and personalized. At the same time, it is important to recognize that technology is not a replacement for human connection and that social support remains essential for mental well-being.

By working together—governments, healthcare providers, schools, employers, and communities—we can create a world where mental health is prioritized and supported, and where individuals have the resources and care they need in order to thrive.

DR. CRANDALL'S AMERICA:
The Mental Health Crisis in the Modern World

Throughout my career, I have witnessed firsthand how mental health struggles have become an epidemic in America. What was once a quiet, often ignored issue has now exploded into a full-blown crisis affecting individuals of all ages, backgrounds, and economic statuses. I've seen how stress, anxiety, depression, and burnout have become normalized, and how the healthcare system often fails to provide the necessary support.

One of my most heartbreaking cases involved a young woman named Rebecca. She was a 23-year-old recent college graduate who came to my office complaining of chest pain and dizziness. She feared she was having a heart attack. After a thorough examination and tests, her heart was perfectly healthy. Instead, what Rebecca was experiencing was severe anxiety, triggered by mounting student loan debt, job insecurity, and social pressures exacerbated by social media. "I feel like I'm always behind, like I'll never catch up," she confided in me. What struck me most was how common her story was—young people burdened with overwhelming pressure and no clear roadmap for how to cope with it.

I've also seen the devastating consequences of untreated depression. A middle-aged man named Mark came to me for routine care, but something in his demeanor seemed off. He admitted he had been struggling with depression for years but never sought help. "Where I come from, you just tough it out," he told me. Unfortunately, the stigma surrounding mental health, especially for men, prevents many from seeking care until it's too late. Mark had turned to alcohol to self-medicate, which only worsened his physical health. After much encouragement, he finally agreed to see a therapist, and over time, I saw him transform—his energy returned, his blood pressure improved, and he reconnected with his family. His story reaffirmed to me that mental health treatment can be life-changing, but only if people feel safe enough to seek help.

The pandemic only magnified these issues. I will never forget treating frontline workers, single parents, and elderly patients who were all facing unprecedented levels of isolation, fear, and loss. Many patients who had never struggled with mental health before began exhibiting signs of severe anxiety, depression, and even PTSD. One elderly patient, Margaret, had lost her husband to COVID-19 and had been living in total isolation for months. "I feel like I have nothing left to live for," she told me. It was one of the most difficult conversations I've had, knowing that beyond medical treatment, what she truly needed was human connection.

However, I have also seen hopeful progress. More people are speaking openly about mental health, and younger generations are advocating for change in ways I never saw early in my career. Workplaces are implementing mental health benefits, schools are teaching mindfulness, and there is growing awareness of the mind-body connection. I worked with one community that created a wellness program combining exercise, nutrition, and group therapy, and the results were astounding— reduced stress levels, better physical health, and stronger social bonds.

Despite these positive shifts, the challenges remain. Access to mental health care is still a significant barrier, especially in rural areas and lower-income communities.

Too many people cannot afford therapy or wait months for an appointment with a psychiatrist. We need systemic changes that prioritize mental well-being as much as physical health.

Through all of this focus, my biggest takeaway has been this: Mental health is not a luxury—it is a necessity. It affects every aspect of our lives, from our relationships to our physical health to our ability to thrive. As a doctor, I have learned that treating the body is only part of the equation. Addressing mental well-being is just as critical, and until our healthcare system recognizes this need fully, we will continue to fall short of truly healing our nation.

R℞ Dr. Crandall's Prescription for Better Mental Health in the Modern World

- ✔ **Create a Daily Mindfulness Practice.** Incorporate meditation, deep breathing, or gratitude exercises into your routine to reduce stress and improve mental clarity.
- ✔ **Recognize the Impact of Digital Overload.** Set boundaries for social media and screen time to prevent information fatigue, anxiety, and negative mental health effects.
- ✔ **Prioritize Work-Life Balance.** Establish clear boundaries between work and personal life to prevent burnout and maintain emotional well-being.
- ✔ **Seek Professional Mental Health Support.** Understand that therapy and counseling are valuable tools, not signs of weakness, and utilize mental health services when needed.
- ✔ **Develop Emotional Intelligence.** Improve self-awareness and interpersonal relationships by actively managing emotions, improving communication, and practicing empathy.

✔ **Engage in Regular Physical Activity for Mental Health Benefits.** Exercise has been shown to reduce depression, anxiety, and stress, making it a crucial tool for overall mental well-being.

✔ **Build a Support Network.** Surround yourself with positive relationships, seek community engagement, and maintain social connections to foster resilience against mental health struggles.

Resources

Volunteering is an excellent way to combat social isolation and improve mental health. Here are two resources that can match you up with places to volunteer in your community.

Volunteer Match
Ways to match your skills and interests with volunteer opportunities in your community (https://www.volunteermatch.org).

Idealist
The largest network of nonprofit organizations offering opportunities to volunteer locally or remotely (https://www.idealist.org/en).

U.S. Department of Health and Human Services
A downloadable guide on the impact of social media on youth mental health, along with topic links (https://www.hhs.gov/surgeongeneral/reports-and-publications/youth-mental-health/social-media/index.html).

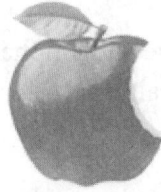

CHAPTER FOURTEEN

AGING AND HEALTH: PREPARING FOR AN AGING POPULATION

As populations around the world grow older, aging has become one of the most pressing public health challenges of the twenty-first century. In the United States, and many other developed nations, people are living longer due to advances in healthcare, nutrition, and technology. By 2030, one in five Americans will be over the age of 65, a demographic shift that presents significant challenges and opportunities for healthcare systems, social services, and communities. This chapter explores the health implications of aging, the social and economic factors that influence the well-being of older adults, and the strategies needed to create age-friendly environments that support healthy aging.

Aging is not just about extending life; it is about ensuring that people can live those extra years in good health. Chronic diseases, mobility issues, cognitive decline, and social isolation are some of the key challenges that older adults face. Addressing these challenges will require a comprehensive approach that integrates healthcare, social services, housing, and community support. Additionally, the chapter will examine the concept of "successful aging," which goes beyond merely surviving into old age and emphasizes maintaining physical, cognitive, and emotional health.

THE HEALTH IMPLICATIONS OF AGING

As people age, they become more susceptible to a variety of health conditions, many of which can impact their quality of life. The most common health challenges faced by older adults include chronic diseases, cognitive decline, mobility issues, and sensory impairments. Understanding these conditions and how they interact is essential for developing strategies to support healthy aging.

Chronic Diseases

Chronic diseases are the leading cause of death and disability among older adults. Conditions such as heart disease, cancer, diabetes, and chronic obstructive pulmonary disease (COPD) are prevalent in the aging population and often require long-term management. According to the Centers for Disease Control and Prevention (CDC), 85% of older adults in the United States have at least one chronic health condition, and 60% have two or more.

Managing chronic diseases in older adults can be challenging because many individuals have multiple conditions that require complex treatment regimens. For example, a person with diabetes may also have hypertension and heart disease, which increases the risk of complications and hospitalizations. Additionally, older adults may experience reduced mobility, making it difficult to engage in regular physical activity, which is a key component of managing chronic diseases.

Effective management of chronic diseases in older adults requires a holistic approach that includes regular medical care, medication management, physical activity, and dietary changes. It also requires coordination between healthcare providers to ensure that treatments for multiple conditions are well-integrated and do not conflict with one another.

Cognitive Decline and Dementia

Cognitive decline is one of the most feared aspects of aging, and it can have a significant impact on an individual's ability to live independently. Age-related cognitive decline can manifest as memory problems, difficulty concentrating, and trouble with decision-making. While some degree of cognitive decline is a normal part of aging, more severe forms, such as Alzheimer's disease and other types of dementia, affect millions of older adults.

Dementia is a progressive condition that impairs cognitive function to the point where it interferes with daily activities. Alzheimer's disease is the most common form of dementia, accounting for 60–80% of cases. In the United States, approximately six million people are living with Alzheimer's, and that number is expected to rise as the population ages. Dementia not only affects the individual but also places a significant burden on caregivers, both emotionally and financially.

While there is currently no cure for Alzheimer's or other forms of dementia, early diagnosis and interventions can help slow the progression of the disease and improve quality of life. Cognitive training, physical activity, and social engagement have been shown to reduce the risk of cognitive decline and improve brain health in older adults. Additionally, medications are available that can help manage symptoms in the early stages of the disease.

Mobility and Falls

Mobility issues are another common challenge for older adults. As people age, they may experience a decline in muscle strength, balance, and coordination, which increases the risk of falls. Falls are a leading cause of injury and hospitalization among older adults, and they can lead to serious complications such as fractures, head injuries, and a loss of independence. According to the CDC, one in four Americans over the age of 65 falls each year, and falls are the leading cause of injury-related deaths among older adults.

Preventing falls requires a combination of strategies, including regular exercise to improve strength and balance, home modifications to reduce fall hazards, and vision and hearing checks to ensure that sensory impairments do not contribute to falls. Additionally, healthcare providers should regularly assess older adults for fall risk and provide interventions as needed.

Sensory Impairments

Hearing and vision impairments are common among older adults and can significantly affect quality of life. Approximately one-third of adults over the age of 65 have some degree of hearing loss, and the prevalence increases with age. Untreated hearing loss is associated with social isolation, depression, and cognitive decline. Similarly, vision problems, such as cataracts, macular degeneration, and glaucoma, can impair an individual's ability to perform daily activities and increase the risk of falls.

Addressing sensory impairments in older adults requires regular screenings and access to assistive devices, such as hearing aids and glasses. However, many older adults do not receive the necessary treatment for these conditions due to cost, lack of awareness, or stigma. Improving access to care and reducing the stigma associated with assistive devices are important steps in supporting healthy aging.

SOCIAL DETERMINANTS OF HEALTH IN AGING

The social determinants of health—conditions in which people are born, grow, live, work, and age—play a significant role in shaping the health outcomes of older adults. Factors such as income, education, housing, and social support can either contribute to or mitigate the challenges associated with aging.

Income and Economic Security

Economic security is a key determinant of health for older adults. Many older individuals rely on fixed incomes from Social Security, pensions, or savings, and financial insecurity can limit their ability to access healthcare, nutritious food, and other essential services. Older adults who live in poverty are at greater risk of poor health outcomes, including chronic diseases, mental health problems, and premature death.

In the United States, disparities in economic security are stark, particularly for women, people of color, and those who have worked in low-wage jobs throughout their lives. For example, women often have lower retirement savings than men due to factors such as the gender pay gap and time taken out of the workforce for caregiving responsibilities. Additionally, Black and Latino older adults are more likely to experience poverty and have less access to resources that support healthy aging.

Addressing the economic challenges faced by older adults will require policies that strengthen retirement security, such as expanding Social Security benefits, increasing access to affordable healthcare, and providing financial support for long-term care services.

Housing and Living Arrangements

Safe and affordable housing is essential for the health and well-being of older adults. Many older individuals prefer to age in place, meaning they wish to remain in their homes and communities as they grow older. However, aging in place can be challenging, particularly for individuals with mobility issues or those living in homes that are not designed to accommodate their needs. Lack of access to transportation, healthcare services, and social activities can contribute to social isolation and poor health outcomes for older adults who live alone.

In addition to aging in place, some older adults live in assisted living facilities, nursing homes, or with family members. These living arrangements can provide additional support but also come with their own challenges. For example, nursing homes have been criticized for providing inadequate care, and many families struggle to afford the high costs of assisted living.

To support healthy aging, communities need to provide a range of housing options that are affordable, accessible, and designed to meet the needs of older adults. This includes retrofitting homes with features such as grab bars, ramps, and widened doorways, as well as developing age-friendly communities with access to healthcare, public transportation, and social services.

Social Support and Isolation

Social support is a critical component of healthy aging. Older adults who have strong social networks, including family, friends, and community connections, are more likely to maintain their mental and physical health as they age. Conversely, social isolation and loneliness are major risk factors for poor health outcomes, including depression, cognitive decline, and premature death.

Unfortunately, many older adults experience social isolation due to factors such as the loss of a spouse, retirement, or mobility issues that limit their ability to participate in social activities. The COVID-19 pandemic exacerbated this problem, as social distancing measures have further limited opportunities for older adults to connect with others.

Addressing social isolation requires a multi-faceted approach that includes creating opportunities for older adults to engage in social activities, providing transportation services, and utilizing technology to connect individuals who are unable to leave their homes. Programs that pair older adults with volunteers, such as phone or virtual companions, can help reduce loneliness and improve mental health.

HEALTHCARE FOR AN AGING POPULATION

As the population ages, healthcare systems will face increasing demand for services related to chronic disease management, long-term care, and end-of-life care. Ensuring that healthcare systems are equipped to meet the needs of older adults is essential for promoting healthy aging and improving quality of life.

Geriatric Care

Geriatric care, which focuses on the health needs of older adults, is an essential component of healthcare systems as populations age. Geriatricians are trained to address the complex and often overlapping health issues that older adults face, including managing multiple chronic conditions, assessing fall risk, and addressing cognitive decline. However, there is currently a shortage of geriatricians in many countries, including the United States, where there are fewer than 7,500 board-certified geriatricians to serve a rapidly growing older population.

Expanding the geriatric workforce will require increased funding for geriatric training programs, as well as incentives to encourage medical students to specialize in geriatrics. Additionally, integrating geriatric care into primary care settings can help ensure that older adults receive the specialized care they need without having to see multiple providers.

Long-Term Care

Long-term care services, which include assistance with activities of daily living (ADLs) such as bathing, dressing, and eating, are critical for older adults who are no longer able to live independently. Long-term care can be provided in nursing homes or assisted living facilities, or through home-based care services. However, the cost of long-term care is often prohibitive, and many families struggle to afford the services their loved ones need.

In the United States, Medicaid is the primary payer for long-term care services, but eligibility is limited to individuals with very low incomes and assets. Expanding access to affordable long-term care services, including home-based care, is essential for supporting older adults who wish to age in place. Additionally, policies that provide financial support for family caregivers, who often bear the brunt of long-term care responsibilities, can help ease the burden on families and improve the quality of care for older adults.

End-of-Life Care

End-of-life care, including palliative care and hospice, is an important aspect of healthcare for older adults. Palliative care focuses on managing symptoms and improving quality of life for individuals with serious illnesses, while hospice provides care and support for individuals who are nearing the end of life. Both types of care emphasize comfort, dignity, and support for patients and their families.

Despite the benefits of palliative and hospice care, many older adults do not receive these services, either because they are unaware of them or are not referred by their healthcare providers. Increasing awareness of end-of-life care options and integrating palliative care into routine healthcare for older adults can improve quality of life and reduce unnecessary hospitalizations.

THE CONCEPT OF SUCCESSFUL AGING

The concept of "successful aging" goes beyond simply living longer; it emphasizes the importance of maintaining physical, cognitive, and emotional health as people age. Successful aging involves staying active, engaged, and socially connected, as well as managing health conditions in a way that allows individuals to maintain their independence and quality of life.

Physical Activity and Exercise

Regular physical activity is one of the most important factors in promoting successful aging. Exercise helps maintain muscle strength, balance, and flexibility, all of which are essential for preventing falls and maintaining mobility. Physical activity is also linked to better cognitive function and mental health, as well as a reduced risk of chronic diseases such as heart disease, diabetes, and osteoporosis.

Older adults should aim to engage in a combination of aerobic exercise, strength training, and balance exercises. Programs such as tai chi, yoga, and water aerobics are particularly beneficial for improving balance and flexibility, while walking, swimming, and cycling can help maintain cardiovascular health.

Cognitive Engagement

Staying mentally active is another key component of successful aging. Cognitive engagement, such as reading, doing puzzles, and learning new skills, can help maintain brain health and reduce the risk of cognitive decline. Social engagement, such as participating in group activities or volunteering, also plays a role in promoting cognitive health.

In addition to these activities, maintaining a healthy diet and getting enough sleep are important for brain health. A diet rich in fruits, vegetables, whole grains, and omega-3 fatty acids has been linked to better cognitive function, while poor sleep has been associated with an increased risk of dementia.

Emotional Well-Being

Emotional well-being is an important aspect of successful aging. Older adults who maintain a positive outlook on life, engage in meaningful activities, and have strong social connections are more likely to experience emotional well-being as they age. However, older adults are also at increased risk for mental health issues such as depression and anxiety, particularly if they are socially isolated or dealing with chronic health conditions.

Addressing mental health in older adults requires providing access to counseling, support groups, and social activities that can help reduce feelings of loneliness and isolation. Additionally, healthcare providers should screen older adults for signs of depression and anxiety and provide appropriate interventions.

CONCLUSION: PREPARING FOR AN AGING POPULATION

As the population continues to age, addressing the health needs of older adults will become increasingly important. Supporting healthy aging requires a comprehensive approach that includes managing chronic diseases, preventing falls and cognitive decline, and addressing the social determinants of health. It also requires expanding access to geriatric care, long-term care services, and end-of-life care.

Creating age-friendly communities, improving access to affordable housing, and providing opportunities for social engagement and physical activity are essential for promoting successful aging. By preparing for the needs of an aging population, society can ensure that older adults are able to live longer, healthier, and more fulfilling lives.

DR. CRANDALL'S AMERICA:
The Challenges of an Aging Population

Throughout my career, I have seen firsthand how the challenges associated with aging have become increasingly complex; while modern medicine has certainly extended life expectancy and improved the quality of life for many individuals, the reality remains that our healthcare system is woefully unprepared to meet the needs of a rapidly aging population, particularly as more Americans are living longer but are not necessarily living healthier. As I sit with elderly patients who struggle with multiple chronic conditions—many of which could have been prevented or better managed earlier in life—I often find myself wondering how our society can do better to provide not only medical care but also dignity, respect, and a sense of purpose to those in their later years.

One of the most heartbreaking cases I encountered was that of Mr. Thomas, an 82-year-old man who had been relatively healthy for most of his life but found himself overwhelmed with a series of debilitating health issues, ranging from heart disease to cognitive decline, which left him unable to care for himself without assistance. His daughter, who had been acting as his primary caregiver, broke down in tears in my office, expressing her exhaustion and frustration, not because she didn't love her father, but because she simply had no support; our system expects family members to shoulder the burden of care without offering adequate resources, financial relief, or guidance on how to navigate the complexities of elder care. I see this scenario repeated over and over again, as adult children struggle to balance their own lives while ensuring their aging parents receive the attention and medical oversight they desperately need.

In another particularly poignant case, I remember Mrs. Rodriguez, a 76-year-old woman who had been widowed for over a decade and had no children to assist her as her health began to decline; she came to my office with uncontrolled diabetes and severe arthritis, yet her biggest concern wasn't her physical ailments but the crushing loneliness she felt on a daily basis. She confided in me that she often went days without speaking to another person, and she only made doctor's appointments just to have some form of human interaction; this, to me, is one of the greatest failures of our healthcare and social support systems, as we have neglected to recognize that aging is not merely a biological process but an emotional and psychological journey that requires as much care as any physical condition.

Despite the many heartbreaking cases I have seen, there are glimmers of hope in communities that have begun prioritizing aging wellness initiatives, and I have had the privilege of working with senior programs that integrate social engagement with medical care, demonstrating that holistic approaches can make an enormous difference in both mental and physical well-being. I recall a local wellness initiative in a small town where the church partnered with a community center to provide daily exercise classes, healthy meal services, and social activities for seniors; I saw individuals who had been struggling with isolation and deteriorating health suddenly regain a sense of purpose, their blood pressure improving, their cognitive function stabilizing, and their emotional well-being transforming simply because they felt valued, engaged, and cared for in a way that extended beyond a prescription bottle or a rushed doctor's visit.

However, for every successful program I have witnessed, there are still too many individuals slipping through the cracks, and I find myself continually frustrated by the lack of comprehensive healthcare planning for the elderly, particularly in lower-income communities where access to even basic geriatric care remains a privilege rather than a guaranteed right. I've had patients ration their medications because their fixed incomes simply didn't allow them to afford both their prescriptions and their groceries; I've had elderly individuals refuse treatment for serious conditions because they were afraid of the medical bills that would follow; I've had families break apart under the weight of caregiving stress because they were left without the resources to properly manage the health needs of their aging loved ones.

I am convinced that until we shift our perspective on aging and begin treating it as a phase of life that requires just as much proactive investment as childhood or middle age, we will continue to see growing numbers of elderly individuals suffer unnecessarily; we must create policies that provide better home healthcare support, expand Medicare coverage for essential services, and incentivize the medical field to train more geriatric specialists, as there are simply not enough physicians dedicated to the unique needs of aging patients. If we do not take action now, we will not only fail the current aging population, but we will also be setting ourselves up for an unsustainable future where aging is synonymous with suffering rather than with wisdom, dignity, and a fulfilling quality of life.

While there are moments where I see progress, and I have certainly encountered families, communities, and organizations that are trying to make a difference, I know that unless we address these systemic issues at a national level, the burden will continue to fall on individuals who are least equipped to handle it; aging should not be an uphill battle against bureaucracy, financial hardship, and loneliness, yet for far too many of my patients, that is exactly what it has become. As a physician, I can provide care, advice, and support, but I know that true change will only come when we, as a society, decide that our elders deserve better—not just in words, but in meaningful actions that reshape the way we approach aging in America.

R℞ Dr. Crandall's Prescription for Aging and Health

✔ **Prioritize Strength and Mobility Training.** Incorporate weight-bearing exercises, stretching, and balance training to maintain muscle mass and flexibility and prevent falls as you age.

✔ **Adopt a Brain-Healthy Lifestyle.** Engage in lifelong learning, puzzles, reading, and social activities to stimulate cognitive function and reduce the risk of dementia and neurodegenerative diseases.

✔ **Plan for Long-Term Healthcare Needs.** Research and prepare for aging-related medical care, including advanced directives, long-term care insurance, and access to geriatric specialists.

✔ **Maintain a Strong Social Network.** Build and sustain relationships with family, friends, and community groups to combat loneliness, which is linked to a decline in mental and physical health in aging populations.

✔ **Monitor Nutritional Needs for Aging.** Adjust dietary habits to include nutrient-dense foods that support bone health, cardiovascular function, and digestion while managing age-related metabolic changes.

✔ **Stay Proactive with Regular Health Screenings.** Schedule age-appropriate screenings for conditions such as osteoporosis, cancer, heart disease, and metabolic disorders to catch potential issues early.

✔ **Embrace Purposeful Aging.** Find new hobbies, volunteer, mentor younger generations, or take on new challenges to maintain a sense of purpose, which has been linked to better overall well-being in older adults.

Resources

Healthy Aging and Dementia: Educational Resources and Tool Kit
Information for people and caregivers on Alzheimer's disease, exercise, social isolation, outreach and more (https://www.nia.nih gov/toolkits).

LongtermCare.gov
A government website providing information on long-term care, including planning. Topics include who needs long-term care, what it will cost, what Medicare, Medicaid and other government programs cover, housing, legal information, and where to get help (https://acl .gov/ltc).

Senior Planet
An AARP-sponsored service providing in-person and online courses including digital technology, exercise, tai chi, storytelling, and more (https://seniorplanet.org).

National Council on Aging
Resources on economic well-being, fall prevention, healthy aging programs, senior centers, and workplace training (www.ncoa.org).

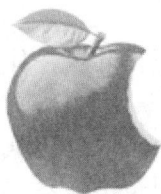

CHAPTER FIFTEEN

CHILD HEALTH: BUILDING A STRONG FOUNDATION

C hildren are the most vulnerable members of society, and their health forms the cornerstone of a nation's future well-being. Ensuring that children have a strong foundation for healthy growth and development is critical not only for their immediate well-being but also for their long-term prospects as adults. Healthy children are more likely to become healthy adults, contributing positively to society. However, across the globe, millions of children face significant health challenges due to factors such as poverty, poor nutrition, lack of access to healthcare, and exposure to environmental hazards.

This chapter will explore the key determinants of child health, including prenatal care, nutrition, access to healthcare, and the importance of early childhood development. We will also examine the leading health issues that children face today, including infectious diseases, chronic conditions, and mental health challenges. Finally, we will discuss the policies and programs that can improve child health outcomes and build a healthier future for all children.

THE FOUNDATIONS OF CHILD HEALTH

The health of a child is shaped by multiple factors, beginning even before birth. A child's well-being is influenced by their genetic makeup, the health and lifestyle of their parents, their physical and social environments, and the care they receive throughout their early years. These early influences can have profound and lasting effects on a child's physical, emotional, and cognitive development.

Prenatal Care and Maternal Health

The foundation for a child's health begins in the womb. Prenatal care and maternal health play critical roles in determining the health outcomes of children. A healthy pregnancy increases the likelihood of a healthy birth, while maternal malnutrition, illness, or substance abuse can lead to complications that affect a child's development before they are even born.

Prenatal care ensures that both the mother and the developing fetus receive regular monitoring and medical support. During pregnancy, healthcare providers monitor the mother's health, screen for potential complications, and provide guidance on nutrition, physical activity, and avoiding harmful substances. Regular prenatal visits can help detect issues such as gestational diabetes, hypertension, or infections that may complicate the pregnancy and lead to poor birth outcomes.

Maternal health is also influenced by social determinants, such as access to healthcare, financial stability, and education. Women living in poverty or in areas with limited healthcare services may be less likely to receive adequate prenatal care, which can contribute to adverse birth outcomes such as preterm birth, low birth weight, and birth defects. Addressing these social determinants of health is crucial for improving maternal and child health outcomes.

Nutrition and Early Childhood Development

Proper nutrition is essential for a child's physical and cognitive development, especially during the critical early years of life. The first 1,000 days—starting from conception through the first two years of life—are particularly important for brain development, immune system function, and overall growth. Children who receive adequate nutrition during this period are more likely to thrive physically, cognitively, and emotionally.

Breastfeeding is considered the best source of nutrition for infants and provides essential antibodies that help protect babies from infections. The World Health Organization (WHO) recommends exclusive breastfeeding for the first six months of life, followed by continued breastfeeding along with the introduction of solid foods. Breastfeeding has been shown to reduce the risk of sudden infant death syndrome (SIDS), gastrointestinal infections, and respiratory illnesses. It also promotes healthy brain development and bonding between mother and child.

For older infants and young children, a balanced diet that includes a variety of fruits, vegetables, grains, proteins, and healthy fats is essential for supporting growth and development. Malnutrition, whether due to undernutrition or overnutrition, can have serious long-term effects on a child's health. Undernutrition can lead to stunting (impaired growth and development) and weakened immune systems, while obesity increases the risk of chronic diseases such as type 2 diabetes, heart disease, and hypertension.

Early Childhood Development

The early years of life are critical for brain development. During this period, a child's brain undergoes rapid growth and forms the neural connections that lay the foundation for cognitive, social, and emotional development. Children who experience nurturing, supportive environments with opportunities for learning and exploration are more likely to develop the skills they need to succeed in school and later in life.

Early childhood development (ECD) programs that focus on cognitive stimulation, emotional support, and social interaction have been shown to improve long-term outcomes for children. For example, high-quality early childhood education programs, such as Head Start in the United States, provide children with early learning experiences that promote cognitive and language development. These programs also support parents by offering resources and guidance on how to foster their children's development at home.

In contrast, children who experience adverse childhood experiences (ACEs), such as abuse, neglect, or exposure to violence, are at higher risk for poor health outcomes later in life. ACEs can disrupt brain development and lead to problems such as learning disabilities, behavioral issues, and mental health disorders. Preventing ACEs and providing support to families in crisis is essential for protecting children's health and well-being.

MAJOR HEALTH ISSUES FACING CHILDREN

While many children in high-income countries grow up in environments that support their health and development, millions of children around the world face significant health challenges. Infectious diseases, chronic conditions, mental health disorders, and environmental hazards are among the leading health issues that affect children today.

Infectious Diseases

Infectious diseases remain a leading cause of morbidity and mortality among children, particularly in low- and middle-income countries.

Despite significant progress in reducing child mortality rates, diseases such as pneumonia, diarrhea, and malaria continue to claim the lives of millions of children each year.

Pneumonia is the leading infectious cause of death in children under five, responsible for approximately 800,000 deaths annually. Many of these deaths are preventable with vaccines, timely treatment, and access to basic healthcare services. Similarly, diarrheal diseases, often caused by contaminated water and poor sanitation, are a major cause of death and illness in young children. Improved access to clean water, sanitation, and vaccines can significantly reduce the burden of these diseases.

Malaria remains a significant threat to children's health in many parts of Africa and Southeast Asia. While efforts to distribute bed nets and provide antimalarial medications have helped reduce malaria-related deaths, the disease continues to pose a serious risk to young children, particularly in rural areas where access to healthcare is limited.

Vaccination has been one of the most successful public health interventions for preventing infectious diseases in children. Vaccines protect against diseases such as measles, polio, and whooping cough, which were once leading causes of child mortality. However, vaccine hesitancy and misinformation continue to pose challenges, leading to outbreaks of preventable diseases in some regions.

Chronic Conditions

While infectious diseases remain a significant concern, chronic conditions are increasingly affecting children, particularly in high-income countries. Childhood obesity, asthma, and type 1 diabetes are among the most common chronic health conditions that impact children's quality of life.

Childhood obesity has reached epidemic proportions in many parts of the world, driven by poor diets, sedentary lifestyles, and an overabundance of processed, calorie-dense foods. Obesity increases the risk of developing chronic conditions such as type 2 diabetes, hypertension, and heart disease, even in childhood. It also has a significant impact on children's mental health, contributing to low self-esteem, anxiety, and depression.

Asthma is another common chronic condition that affects millions of children worldwide. Asthma is characterized by inflammation of the airways, which leads to difficulty breathing, coughing, and wheezing. Environmental factors such as air pollution, exposure to tobacco smoke, and allergens can trigger asthma attacks, making it a major public health concern, particularly in urban areas.

Type 1 diabetes, an autoimmune condition in which the body does not produce insulin, is also on the rise among children. Managing type 1 diabetes requires lifelong monitoring of blood sugar levels, insulin administration, and dietary management. While children with type 1 diabetes can live healthy, active lives with proper management, the condition can have a significant impact on daily life and increase the risk of complications.

Mental Health

Mental health disorders in children are often overlooked, but they are becoming increasingly prevalent in today's society. Anxiety, depression, and behavioral disorders are among the most common mental health issues affecting children and adolescents. Left untreated, these conditions can have serious consequences for a child's development, academic performance, and overall well-being.

Anxiety disorders are the most common mental health conditions among children and adolescents, affecting approximately one in eight children. Anxiety can manifest in various ways, including excessive worrying, social withdrawal, and physical symptoms such as headaches and stomachaches. Depression is also a growing concern among children, particularly adolescents. Depression in children often presents as irritability, sadness, or a lack of interest in activities they once enjoyed.

Behavioral disorders, such as attention-deficit/hyperactivity disorder (ADHD) and oppositional defiant disorder (ODD), can also have a significant impact on a child's ability to succeed in school and interact with peers. Children with behavioral disorders may struggle with impulse control, following rules, and maintaining relationships, which can lead to difficulties in school and social settings.

Early intervention is critical for addressing mental health issues in children. Schools play a key role in identifying children who may be struggling with mental health problems and providing access to counseling, support groups, and other resources. Additionally, healthcare providers should screen children for mental health issues during routine check-ups and refer them to appropriate services as needed.

ENVIRONMENTAL FACTORS AND CHILD HEALTH

Children are particularly vulnerable to environmental hazards, such as air pollution, lead exposure, and unsafe water. These environmental factors can have long-term effects on a child's health, leading to respiratory problems, developmental delays, and chronic conditions.

Air Pollution

Air pollution is a major public health concern, particularly in urban areas where children are exposed to high levels of particulate matter, nitrogen dioxide, and other pollutants. Exposure to air pollution has been linked to respiratory problems such as asthma, bronchitis, and pneumonia. Children are more susceptible to the effects of air pollution because their lungs are still developing, and they tend to spend more time outdoors.

Reducing air pollution requires a combination of policy interventions, such as reducing emissions from vehicles and industrial sources, and community-level actions, such as increasing green spaces and promoting active transportation. Schools and childcare centers should be located away from major highways and industrial areas to minimize children's exposure to harmful pollutants.

Lead Exposure

Lead exposure is another significant environmental health issue for children. Lead is a toxic metal that can cause developmental delays, learning disabilities, and behavioral problems. Children are most commonly exposed to lead through lead-based paint, contaminated soil, and old plumbing systems. Although lead has been banned from use in paint and gasoline in many countries, millions of children are still exposed to dangerous levels of lead, particularly in older homes and in low-income communities.

Preventing lead exposure requires regular testing of homes, schools, and childcare centers for lead contamination, as well as public education campaigns to raise awareness about the dangers of lead. Additionally, policies that support the removal of lead from the environment, such as replacing lead pipes and remediating contaminated soil, are essential for protecting children from this harmful substance.

Safe Water and Sanitation

Access to clean water and sanitation is essential for protecting children from waterborne diseases and promoting overall health. In many parts of the world, children are exposed to contaminated water and poor sanitation, which can lead to diarrheal diseases, malnutrition, and stunting. The lack of access to clean water and sanitation disproportionately affects children in low-income and rural areas.

Improving access to clean water and sanitation requires investment in infrastructure, including building safe water systems and latrines in schools and communities. Education programs that teach children and families about proper hygiene practices, such as handwashing with soap, can also help reduce the spread of infectious diseases.

POLICIES AND PROGRAMS TO IMPROVE CHILD HEALTH

Addressing the health challenges faced by children requires comprehensive policies and programs that support their physical, emotional, and cognitive development. Governments, healthcare systems, schools, and communities all play roles in promoting child health and ensuring that every child has the opportunity to thrive.

Access to Healthcare

Ensuring that children have access to healthcare is essential for preventing and treating illness, promoting healthy development, and reducing health disparities. In the United States, programs such as Medicaid and the Children's Health Insurance Program (CHIP) provide health coverage to millions of low-income children. Expanding access to these programs and reducing barriers to care, such as transportation problems and language barriers, can help ensure that all children receive the healthcare services they need.

Vaccination Programs

Vaccination programs are one of the most effective ways to protect children from infectious diseases. Governments and public health organizations should continue to promote vaccine coverage, particularly in underserved and remote areas. Public education campaigns that address vaccine hesitancy and misinformation are also essential for ensuring high vaccination rates.

Early Childhood Education and Care

High-quality early childhood education programs, such as Head Start, play a critical role in promoting child health and development. These programs provide children with early learning experiences, access to healthcare services, and nutritious meals. Expanding access to early childhood education, particularly in low-income communities, can help reduce disparities in child health outcomes and improve long-term success.

Nutrition Programs

Programs such as the Special Supplemental Nutrition Program for Women, Infants, and Children (WIC) and the National School Lunch Program (NSLP) provide essential nutrition support to low-income children. These programs help ensure that children receive the healthy foods they need for proper growth and development. Expanding access to these programs and promoting nutrition education can help reduce rates of malnutrition and obesity in children.

CONCLUSION: BUILDING A HEALTHY FUTURE FOR CHILDREN

Children are the foundation of society, and investing in their health is an investment in the future. By addressing the social, economic, and environmental factors that influence child health, we can create a world where every child has the opportunity to grow up healthy and thrive. Ensuring access to healthcare, proper nutrition, early childhood education, and safe environments is essential for promoting the physical, cognitive, and emotional well-being of children.

Governments, communities, healthcare providers, and families must work together to create policies and programs that support children's health and development. By building a strong foundation for children's health, we can help them grow into healthy, productive adults who contribute to the well-being of society as a whole.

DR. CRANDALL'S AMERICA:
The Challenges and Hope for Children's Health

Throughout my career, I have seen how the health of our children is a direct reflection of the priorities we set as a society. In recent years, I have become increasingly alarmed at the rise in chronic illnesses among children, the decline in physical activity, and the overwhelming impact of poor nutrition, stress, and screen time on their well-being. While modern medicine has given us incredible tools to combat disease, the reality is that too many children are growing up in environments that set them up for a lifetime of health struggles.

One of the most heartbreaking cases I encountered was that of Jake, an 11-year-old boy who came to my office struggling with obesity and early signs of type 2 diabetes. His mother was in tears, explaining how she worked multiple jobs and had little time to cook, often relying on fast food and processed meals. "I just don't know how to fix this," she said. Jake had already developed high blood pressure and was struggling with low self-esteem due to bullying at school. The hardest part of cases like Jake's is that they are preventable—if we prioritize childhood nutrition, food education, and accessible, affordable healthy options, children like him won't have to suffer.

Another case that has stayed with me is that of Emily, a six-year-old girl who had been diagnosed with severe anxiety. Her parents were well-meaning but had unknowingly contributed to her stress by overloading her with extracurricular activities, excessive screen time, and a lack of unstructured play. "She's always tired, she worries about everything, and she barely sleeps," her father admitted. Emily's story reflects a disturbing trend I have seen in children—many are overstimulated, under-rested, and facing levels of stress that were once considered adult problems. Instead of childhood being a time of exploration, joy, and creativity, many kids are burdened with unrealistic academic and social pressures that take a toll on their mental and physical health.

I have also treated children suffering from preventable illnesses due to a lack of access to healthcare. One heartbreaking case was Miguel, a toddler who developed severe respiratory issues because his family lived in substandard housing with mold and pollution exposure. His parents worked hard but couldn't afford better living conditions. "We take him to the emergency room when it gets bad, but we can't afford specialists," his mother told me. The reality is that children from lower-income families are far more likely to experience chronic illnesses due to poor environmental conditions, inadequate nutrition, and delayed medical care. This is a failure of the system, not the parents.

Despite these challenges, I have also seen hopeful progress. In one community, a local school implemented a wellness program that included healthier school lunches, daily physical activity, and mental health education. I witnessed a remarkable shift in students' energy levels, concentration, and overall well-being. One young girl, previously lethargic and struggling with obesity, proudly told me, "I love the new lunches, and I feel so much better in gym class!" Small changes, when implemented thoughtfully and consistently, can have a profound impact on children's health.

I've also been inspired by parents and communities taking matters into their own hands. I worked with a group of mothers who started a weekend farmers' market near their children's school, ensuring that families had access to fresh fruits and vegetables. I've seen teachers incorporate mindfulness practices into their classrooms, helping kids learn how to manage stress and focus better. I've met pediatricians who push for policy changes to eliminate junk food marketing aimed at kids. These efforts give me hope that positive change is possible if we prioritize children's well-being at every level—at home, in schools, and through public policy.

Yet, there is still so much more to be done. Childhood should be a time of growth, play, and discovery, not of chronic illness, anxiety, and poor health habits that follow kids into adulthood. We need to address the root causes—nutritional education, mental health support, safe environments, and access to quality healthcare—rather than just treating the symptoms.

As a doctor, I can guide individual families, but I know that systemic change is needed to truly reverse the health crisis affecting our children. Every child deserves the chance to grow up healthy, active, and resilient. The question is: Are we willing to fight for their future? Because if we don't, we will be condemning an entire generation to a lifetime of preventable health struggles. The time to act is now.

R℞ Dr. Crandall's Prescription for Child Health

✔ **Establish Healthy Eating Habits Early.** Introduce children to a variety of whole, nutrient-dense foods from a young age to shape lifelong healthy eating behaviors.

✔ **Encourage Active Play and Movement.** Promote outdoor activities, sports, and unstructured play to support physical development and prevent sedentary lifestyles.

✔ **Prioritize Quality Sleep for Growth and Development.** Ensure children get adequate sleep based on their age, as sleep is essential for brain development, immune function, and emotional well-being.

✔ **Limit Screen Time and Promote Mental Stimulation.** Reduce exposure to excessive screen time and encourage reading, creative play, and problem-solving activities to support cognitive growth.

✔ **Teach Emotional Resilience and Coping Skills.** Help children manage stress and emotions through open communication, mindfulness techniques, and positive reinforcement.

✔ **Stay Consistent with Pediatric Check-Ups and Vaccinations.** Monitor developmental milestones, ensure timely vaccinations, and seek preventive healthcare to support long-term well-being.

✔ **Model Healthy Behaviors as a Parent or Caregiver.** Set a positive example by practicing healthy eating, regular exercise, and stress management, as children learn by observing adult behavior.

Resources

Academy of Nutrition and Dietetics Foundation
Toolkits and presentations designed to help parents and teens understand nutrition. Resources include workshops on cooking, smart shopping, and balanced eating (https://www.eatright foundation.org/resources/kids-eat-right).

American Academy of Child and Adolescent Psychiatry (AACAP)
Good screen habits, including when to turn off screens, parental controls, and how to avoid using screens as a substitute for good parenting, are covered (https://www.aacap.org/AACAP/Families_ and_Youth/Facts_for_Families/FFF-Guide/Children-And -Watching-TV-054).

Centers for Disease Control and Prevention (CDC)
Parenting tips for infants, emphasizing self-care for parents and strategies to support your baby's development (https://www.cdc.gov/ child-development/positive-parenting-tips/infants.html).

Centers for Disease Control and Prevention (CDC)
A comprehensive chart of recommended vaccines for children from birth through 18 years old (https://www.cdc.gov/vaccines-children/ schedules/index.html).

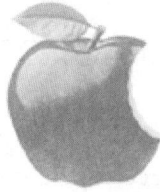

CHAPTER SIXTEEN

HEALTH AND THE ECONOMY: INVESTING IN WELL-BEING

Health and the economy are inextricably linked. A healthy population is fundamental to economic growth, productivity, and social stability. Conversely, poor health undermines economic progress, strains public resources, and exacerbates inequality. The COVID-19 pandemic provided a stark reminder of this connection, as nations around the world grappled with the dual crises of public health and economic downturns. But beyond crises, the relationship between health and economic prosperity operates continuously, shaping the trajectory of nations and communities.

Investing in health is one of the most effective strategies for fostering economic resilience and long-term growth. This chapter will explore the economic implications of health, the cost of poor health, and the benefits of investing in healthcare systems, public health infrastructure, and preventive care. It will also examine how health inequities contribute to economic disparities and what governments, businesses, and communities can do to prioritize well-being as an essential pillar of economic development.

THE ECONOMIC IMPACT OF HEALTH

Health influences the economy in multiple ways, from the productivity of the workforce to the cost of healthcare and social services. A population's overall health affects economic output, income levels, and the sustainability of social safety nets. Healthy individuals are more productive, take fewer sick days, and are better able to contribute to society. In contrast, poor health limits individuals' ability to work, increases absenteeism, and reduces workforce participation, all of which hinder economic growth.

Productivity and Workforce Participation

A healthy workforce is essential for economic productivity. When individuals are in good health, they are more likely to participate in the labor market, work efficiently, and maintain stable employment. Chronic illnesses, disabilities, and mental health disorders can reduce an individual's ability to work, leading to decreased productivity and economic losses.

For example, chronic diseases such as heart disease, diabetes, and respiratory illnesses are leading causes of disability in the United States and other high-income countries. These conditions often require long-term treatment and management, resulting in lost workdays, decreased performance, and early retirement. According to the Centers for Disease Control and Prevention (CDC), productivity losses due to chronic health conditions cost U.S. employers billions of dollars each year. In addition, chronic diseases can force individuals to leave the workforce prematurely, reducing the overall size of the labor force and increasing the economic burden on social welfare programs.

Mental health disorders also have a significant impact on workforce participation. Depression, anxiety, and stress-related conditions are among the leading causes of disability worldwide.

These mental health challenges not only affect individuals' ability to perform their jobs but also lead to higher rates of absenteeism and presenteeism—when employees are physically present but unable to work effectively due to health issues. According to the World Health Organization (WHO), the global economy loses an estimated $1 trillion each year due to depression and anxiety.

Workplace health initiatives that promote mental and physical well-being can have a positive impact on productivity and reduce the economic burden of poor health. Employers that invest in employee wellness programs, mental health resources, and preventive care can reduce absenteeism, improve job satisfaction, and increase overall productivity. Studies have shown that companies with robust employee wellness programs often see a return on investment in the form of reduced healthcare costs and improved employee performance.

Healthcare Costs and Public Expenditure

The cost of healthcare is another significant factor in the relationship between health and the economy. In countries with high healthcare expenditures, such as the United States, the rising cost of medical care places a burden on both individuals and governments. High healthcare costs can lead to economic strain, as governments must allocate large portions of their budgets to healthcare spending, leaving fewer resources available for other critical areas such as education, infrastructure, and social services.

In the United States, healthcare spending accounts for nearly 18% of gross domestic product (GDP), the highest percentage of any industrialized nation. Despite this high level of spending, the United States has poorer health outcomes compared to many countries that spend significantly less on healthcare. This highlights the inefficiency of the American healthcare system, where costs are driven by factors such as high drug prices, administrative overhead, and fragmented care. The economic burden of healthcare spending is felt by individuals, businesses, and the government, with many Americans facing financial hardship due to medical bills.

In addition to the direct costs of healthcare, poor health leads to indirect costs for the economy, including lost productivity, lower tax revenues, and higher social welfare expenditures. For example, individuals who are unable to work due to chronic health conditions may require government assistance, such as disability benefits or unemployment insurance. These costs can add up over time, placing additional strain on public resources.

Health Inequities and Economic Disparities

Health inequities—differences in health outcomes that are closely linked to social, economic, and environmental factors—exacerbate economic disparities within societies. Low-income individuals and marginalized communities are more likely to experience poor health due to limited access to healthcare, unhealthy living conditions, and the social determinants of health, such as poverty, education, and housing.

Health disparities have a ripple effect on the economy, as individuals in poor health are less likely to participate fully in the workforce, leading to lower earnings and reduced economic mobility. For example, people living in low-income neighborhoods often face higher rates of chronic diseases such as diabetes and hypertension, which can limit their ability to work and contribute to economic productivity. In turn, this reduces tax revenues and increases demand for public services, such as healthcare and social assistance programs.

Addressing health inequities is not only a moral imperative but also an economic necessity. By improving access to healthcare, addressing social determinants of health, and reducing disparities in health outcomes, governments and communities can promote economic growth and reduce poverty. Health equity ensures that all individuals, regardless of their background or circumstances, have the opportunity to live healthy, productive lives and contribute to society.

THE COST OF POOR HEALTH

The cost of poor health is substantial, both for individuals and society as a whole. When people are in poor health, they are more likely to require medical care, lose income due to inability to work, and depend on social services for support. These costs accumulate over time, leading to a cycle of poverty and poor health that is difficult to break.

Personal Financial Burden

For individuals, poor health can be financially devastating. Medical bills, lost wages, and the cost of long-term care can lead to financial hardship, debt, and even bankruptcy. In the United States, medical debt is one of the leading causes of bankruptcy, with millions of people struggling to pay for the healthcare they need.

The financial burden of healthcare disproportionately affects low-income individuals, who are less likely to have health insurance and more likely to face high out-of-pocket costs. Even individuals with health insurance may struggle to afford care, as high deductibles, co-pays, and uncovered services can add up quickly. This financial strain can lead to delays in seeking care or forgoing necessary treatment altogether, further worsening health outcomes.

In countries with universal healthcare systems, individuals are protected from the financial burden of medical care, but poor health can still result in lost income and reduced economic mobility. For example, individuals who must take extended time off work due to illness or injury may face reduced earnings and career advancement opportunities.

The Impact on Social Services

Poor health also places a burden on social services, including healthcare, disability benefits, and unemployment insurance. Governments must allocate significant resources to support individuals who are unable to work due to health conditions, which can strain public budgets and reduce the availability of resources for other social programs.

In addition, poor health can lead to increased demand for long-term care services, such as nursing homes, home health aides, and rehabilitation facilities. The cost of long-term care is often prohibitively expensive, and many individuals rely on government programs, such as Medicaid in the United States, to cover these costs. As the population ages, the demand for long-term care is expected to increase, placing additional pressure on public resources.

The Societal Costs of Poor Health

The societal costs of poor health extend beyond the direct financial impact on individuals and governments. Poor health contributes to social inequality, limits economic growth, and reduces overall quality of life. In communities where poor health is prevalent, there is often a cycle of poverty and disadvantage that is difficult to break.

For example, children growing up in poverty are more likely to experience poor health due to factors such as inadequate nutrition, exposure to environmental hazards, and limited access to healthcare. These early health disparities can have long-term consequences, affecting educational attainment, workforce participation, and economic mobility. By addressing the root causes of poor health, society can reduce the long-term economic costs of health disparities and promote greater social equity.

THE BENEFITS OF INVESTING IN HEALTH

Investing in health is one of the most effective strategies for promoting economic growth, reducing poverty, and improving quality of life. By prioritizing healthcare, public health infrastructure, and preventive care, governments and businesses can create healthier, more productive populations and build resilient economies.

Preventive Care and Health Promotion

One of the most cost-effective ways to improve health outcomes and reduce healthcare costs is through preventive care and health promotion. Preventive care includes services such as vaccinations, screenings, and health education that help individuals identify and address health risks before they become serious problems.

For example, vaccinations prevent the spread of infectious diseases, reducing the need for expensive treatments and hospitalizations. Similarly, early detection of chronic diseases, such as cancer or diabetes, through screenings can lead to more effective and less costly treatment. Investing in preventive care not only improves individual health but also reduces the overall burden on healthcare systems.

Health promotion initiatives, such as public health campaigns that encourage healthy eating, physical activity, and smoking cessation, can also have a significant impact on population health. By promoting healthy behaviors, governments and organizations can reduce the prevalence of chronic diseases and improve quality of life. In turn, healthier populations are more productive, contributing to economic growth and reducing healthcare expenditures. For example, a healthier workforce means fewer sick days, lower insurance claims, and higher productivity. When governments prioritize and invest in preventive health measures, they are not only improving lives but also building a more sustainable and cost-effective healthcare system.

Moreover, community-based interventions—such as school health programs, workplace wellness initiatives, and faith-based health education—can be leveraged to reach broader populations with limited access to traditional care. These programs have the power to instill lifelong habits, particularly when started early or reinforced regularly. The return on investment in prevention is clear: every dollar spent on preventive services yields significant savings in avoided medical costs down the line.

Unfortunately, preventive care is often underutilized in the current U.S. healthcare model, which remains heavily focused on treatment rather than prevention. Many insurance providers still allocate limited funding to routine screenings or lifestyle counseling, and public health departments are often underfunded. Shifting the national focus toward prevention—by incentivizing regular check-ups, funding public health campaigns, and integrating preventive services into primary care—will be key to reversing America's health crisis.

CONCLUSION: INVESTING IN WELL-BEING

If we are to make America healthy again, we must stop reacting to disease and start preventing it. Prevention is not just a medical issue—it's an economic and social imperative. Individuals, families, communities, and policymakers must all work together to prioritize health before illness strikes. When we empower people to stay well, we reduce suffering, save lives, and ensure a brighter future for generations to come.

DR. CRANDALL'S AMERICA:
The Cost of Health and the Economy

Throughout my career, I have seen the direct link between financial stability and health. It has become increasingly clear that economic struggles are one of the biggest barriers to well-being in America. I have treated countless patients who delay necessary care, ration medications, or avoid preventive screenings simply because they cannot afford them. As a doctor, it is heartbreaking to know that many of the conditions I see could have been prevented or managed if my patients had had access to the resources they needed.

One of the most devastating cases I have encountered was that of James, a 55-year-old man who suffered a massive heart attack. When I reviewed his history, I discovered that he had been experiencing chest pain for months but never sought medical attention. "I didn't want to rack up more bills," he admitted from his hospital bed. James, like many hardworking Americans, had a job that didn't provide adequate health insurance. His heart attack could have been prevented with routine check-ups and cholesterol management, but the financial burden of medical visits kept him from seeking care.

Then there was Diane, a single mother of two, who struggled to afford her insulin. Despite working full-time, her employer's health plan had high deductibles, leaving her to pay hundreds of dollars a month for the medication that kept her alive. "I try to stretch it out," she told me, referring to taking lower doses than prescribed to make her supply last longer. This is a dangerous and all-too-common practice among diabetics who cannot afford their medications. No one should have to choose between feeding their children and managing a chronic illness.

I have also treated patients who are trapped in cycles of poverty-related illness. One example is Ricardo, a young man in his 30s who developed chronic back pain from years of physically demanding labor. Without paid sick leave, he continued working through the pain until his condition became debilitating. When he finally sought treatment, he needed surgery and months of rehabilitation, which left him unemployed. "If I had been able to rest or get therapy earlier, maybe I wouldn't be in this position," he told me. His story highlights the economic consequences of neglecting preventive care—both for individuals and for society as a whole.

But I have also seen glimmers of hope. In a few communities, I have worked with programs that offer free preventive screenings, affordable prescription plans, and financial literacy courses for managing healthcare expenses. One such program helped a patient named Linda, who had been skipping doctor visits because of cost concerns. With financial assistance and guidance, she was able to receive regular check-ups and make lifestyle changes that reversed her prediabetes. "I never thought I'd have control over my health like this," she said.

Employer wellness programs have also made a difference for some patients. I treated an office worker named Steve who lost 40 pounds and lowered his blood pressure after his company introduced an incentivized health initiative. He had access to gym memberships, healthier cafeteria options, and regular health assessments—all at no extra cost to him. "Having these resources at work changed my life," he told me.

Despite these positive efforts, the economic burden of healthcare in America remains overwhelming for too many people. I have watched as insurance premiums, medication prices, and hospital bills continue to rise, pushing even middle-class families into medical debt. The reality is that the United States spends more on healthcare than any other developed nation, yet our health outcomes are worse in many areas. We have built a system that treats disease rather than preventing it, and the financial consequences are devastating.

As a doctor, I do everything I can to help my patients navigate these challenges, but I know that real solutions require systemic change. We need policies that prioritize preventive care, regulate medication prices, and support working families with affordable healthcare options. Until we invest in well-being at both the individual and societal levels, we will continue to see the consequences of economic inequality manifest in our healthcare system.

The question we must ask ourselves is: How much longer can we afford to ignore the connection between health and the economy? Because every time someone like James delays care, or Diane rations her insulin, or Ricardo works himself into disability, we all pay the price. The time to invest in well-being is now.

R℞ Dr. Crandall's Prescription for a Healthy Economy and Investing in Well-Being

✔ **View Health as a Long-Term Investment.** Prioritize spending on nutritious food, preventive care, and fitness rather than treating health as an afterthought or expense only when illness arises.

✔ **Budget for Preventive Healthcare.** Allocate funds for regular check-ups, dental cleanings, and mental health support, which can prevent costly medical emergencies down the road.

✔ **Advocate for Employer-Sponsored Wellness Programs.** Encourage workplaces to offer health benefits like gym memberships, mental health support, and flexible work schedules to reduce stress and improve productivity.

✔ **Support Policies That Prioritize Public Health.** Vote for initiatives that increase healthcare access, regulate harmful food industries, and promote healthier economic structures that support well-being.

✔ **Choose Cost-Effective, Healthier Alternatives.** Opt for home-cooked meals over fast food, use public parks for exercise instead of expensive gym memberships, and explore affordable community health resources.

✔ **Understand the Connection Between Financial Stability and Health.** Reduce stress-related illnesses by improving financial literacy, saving for medical expenses, and making informed economic decisions.

✔ **Encourage Businesses to Promote Health-Conscious Practices.** Support companies that prioritize ethical food sourcing, fair labor practices, and environmentally sustainable business models that contribute to public well-being.

Resources

Centers for Disease Control and Prevention (CDC)
Resources for improving the quality of life for U.S. workers, including how to create a workplace health program (https://www.cdc.gov/workplace-health-promotion/php/model/index.html).

U.S. Office of Personnel Management (OPM)
Information on Health Savings Accounts, including who qualifies, how to use them, and how to list them on your tax return. Includes a health savings plan worksheet (https://www.opm.gov/healthcare-insurance/healthcare/health-savings-accounts/health-savings-account).

Society for Human Resource Management (SHRM)
Steps to establish a workplace wellness program, including how to assess employee wellness needs and designing programs that align with organizational goals (https://www.shrm.org/topics-tools/tools/how-to-guides/how-to-establish-design-wellness-program).

HRSA Health Center Locator
An easy-to-use tool to locate your local community health center anywhere in the United States (https://findahealthcenter.hrsa.gov).

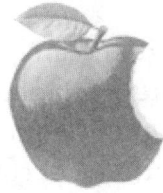

CHAPTER SEVENTEEN

THE ROLE OF FAITH, WORSHIP, AND THE CHURCH IN MAKING AMERICA'S SMALL TOWNS AND BIG CITIES HEALTHY AGAIN

Religious institutions have long been pillars of community life, serving as spiritual and social hubs, particularly in small towns and inner cities. The church and synagogue have played crucial roles in offering support, fostering unity, and providing services to their congregants and the broader community. In a time when America faces significant health challenges, including the rise of chronic diseases, mental health crises, and health inequities, these faith-based institutions can be vital agents in promoting health and wellness. In small towns and inner cities, where healthcare access is often limited and social support systems strained, religious institutions can step in to fill gaps and create lasting impacts on individual and community health.

This chapter will explore the unique role that churches and synagogues can play in improving health outcomes in small towns and inner cities. We will examine the health challenges these communities face, the historical and contemporary contributions of religious institutions to public health, and strategies faith-based organizations can use to promote physical, mental, and spiritual well-being. Through partnerships, advocacy, and direct health services, these institutions can lead the way in making America healthy again.

HEALTH CHALLENGES IN SMALL TOWNS AND INNER CITIES

Both small towns and inner cities face distinct but overlapping health challenges. These areas are often underserved by healthcare systems, lacking sufficient access to medical care, mental health services, and resources that support healthy living. Additionally, socioeconomic factors, such as poverty, unemployment, and housing insecurity, further exacerbate health disparities.

Small Towns

In rural America, small towns often face a shortage of healthcare providers and facilities. Hospitals and clinics are scarce, and residents may have to travel long distances to receive medical care. Rural populations tend to have higher rates of chronic conditions such as diabetes, heart disease, and obesity, and are often underserved in terms of mental health care. According to the National Rural Health Association, rural Americans are more likely to experience higher rates of premature death from preventable conditions due to a lack of timely care and health education.

Compounding these issues is the challenge of isolation. The lack of public transportation, lower population densities, and fewer opportunities for social engagement can lead to higher levels of social isolation and loneliness, which are known risk factors for mental health conditions such as depression and anxiety. Churches and synagogues in these areas can play a vital role in fostering community connections and providing health services.

Inner Cities

Inner-city areas, particularly those with large minority populations, face their own set of health challenges. Many residents live in food deserts—areas where access to fresh, healthy food is limited, leading to poor nutrition and high rates of obesity and diet-related diseases. Inner-city residents are also more likely to be exposed to environmental hazards, such as air pollution and unsafe housing conditions, which contribute to respiratory illnesses and other health issues.

Mental health problems, including anxiety, depression, and trauma, are prevalent in inner cities, often exacerbated by poverty, violence, and unstable housing. Despite the high need for mental health services, many inner-city residents face barriers to accessing care, such as high costs, lack of insurance, and stigma. Additionally, healthcare facilities in inner cities are often overwhelmed, underfunded, and inaccessible to many who need them.

Churches and synagogues in these areas can serve as safe havens, providing not only spiritual support but also practical health services and advocacy for social change. These institutions have a long history of standing up for the most vulnerable members of society, and today, they can use their influence to tackle the root causes of health disparities in inner cities.

THE HISTORICAL ROLE OF CHURCHES AND SYNAGOGUES IN HEALTH PROMOTION

Historically, religious institutions have been central to health promotion, particularly in underserved communities. Churches and synagogues have provided healthcare services, supported public health initiatives, and advocated for social justice, often filling the gaps left by public health systems.

Churches

Christian churches, particularly in African American communities, have long been involved in addressing health disparities. During the civil rights movement, Black churches provided health services to underserved communities, often offering medical care, vaccinations, and health education. They were instrumental in raising awareness about health risks, promoting preventive care, and advocating for equitable healthcare access.

In small towns, churches often provided the first and only healthcare services. Many rural churches established health clinics and hospitals, staffed by church members and volunteers, to serve populations that had little access to formal medical care. The influence of religious hospitals continues today, with many Catholic and Protestant health institutions providing care to underserved populations.

Synagogues

Jewish synagogues have also played a key role in promoting health and social justice, particularly in urban areas. Synagogues in immigrant communities during the late 19th and early 20th centuries offered health services to newly arrived Jewish immigrants, many of whom lived in poverty and had limited access to healthcare. These synagogues provided vaccinations, medical checkups, and health education, often partnering with local charities and Jewish organizations to improve the health of their communities.

Jewish ethics strongly emphasize the concept of *pikuach nefesh*— the preservation of human life—which has guided the involvement of Jewish institutions in healthcare and social services. Synagogues continue to be active in public health advocacy, supporting initiatives to expand healthcare access, reduce poverty, and combat food insecurity.

THE CONTEMPORARY ROLE OF CHURCHES AND SYNAGOGUES IN PROMOTING HEALTH

Today, churches and synagogues remain vital institutions in both small towns and inner cities. As community hubs, they are uniquely positioned to promote health and wellness, provide social support, and advocate for policies that improve the well-being of their congregants and communities. Below are several key roles that religious institutions can play in promoting health.

Health Education and Preventive Care

Churches and synagogues can play a key role in providing health education and promoting preventive care, particularly in communities where access to healthcare services is limited. Many congregants turn to their religious leaders for guidance on health issues, and churches and synagogues can use this trust to promote healthy behaviors.

Faith-based health ministries can organize workshops on topics such as nutrition, exercise, chronic disease prevention, and mental health awareness. These programs can educate community members on the importance of early detection and regular medical checkups, helping to reduce the incidence of preventable diseases.

For example, churches and synagogues can partner with local healthcare providers to offer free health screenings for conditions such as high blood pressure, diabetes, and cholesterol. These screenings can help identify health risks early, allowing individuals to seek treatment before conditions worsen. In rural areas, mobile health clinics can partner with churches to provide medical services directly to residents who may otherwise have difficulty accessing care.

Mental Health Support

Mental health issues are pervasive in both small towns and inner cities, yet many individuals do not seek help due to stigma, lack of resources, or distrust of medical institutions. Churches and synagogues, as trusted institutions, can provide a supportive environment for individuals struggling with mental health challenges. Faith leaders can offer pastoral counseling and spiritual guidance to those in need, while also encouraging congregants to seek professional mental health services when appropriate.

Religious institutions can also offer mental health workshops and support groups, creating spaces for individuals to talk openly about their struggles without fear of judgment. For example, a church might host a support group for individuals dealing with grief, addiction, or depression, offering both spiritual support and practical resources. Synagogues can also partner with mental health organizations to provide education on mental health issues and reduce the stigma associated with seeking help.

Addressing Food Insecurity

In both small towns and inner cities, food insecurity is a major health challenge. Churches and synagogues can play a critical role in addressing this issue by organizing food drives, running food pantries, and supporting community gardens. These programs not only provide immediate relief to families in need but also promote long-term health by ensuring that individuals have access to nutritious, fresh foods.

In inner cities, where many residents live in food deserts, religious institutions can advocate for policies that increase access to healthy foods, such as the establishment of farmers' markets or subsidies for fresh produce. They can also partner with local businesses and nonprofits to distribute healthy meals to low-income families and offer cooking classes that teach congregants how to prepare nutritious meals on a budget.

Advocacy for Health Equity

Churches and synagogues have a long history of advocating for social justice, and this role extends to the fight for health equity. By addressing the social determinants of health—such as poverty, education, housing, and access to healthcare—religious institutions can help reduce health disparities in both small towns and inner cities.

Religious leaders can use their influence to advocate for policies that improve healthcare access, increase funding for public health programs, and address the root causes of health inequities. For example, churches and synagogues can support local and national campaigns to expand Medicaid, increase funding for mental health services, or reduce environmental hazards in low-income neighborhoods.

In addition to policy advocacy, religious institutions can work to break down barriers to healthcare by providing transportation to medical appointments, helping congregants navigate health insurance, and connecting individuals with community resources that can improve their health and well-being.

FAITH-BASED HEALTH INITIATIVES: SUCCESSFUL EXAMPLES

There are already many successful faith-based health initiatives that demonstrate the potential for churches and synagogues to make a meaningful impact on public health.

Health Ministries in Churches

Many churches have established health ministries that focus on promoting physical and mental health within their congregations. These ministries often organize health fairs, offer screenings for common health conditions, and provide education on nutrition, exercise, and disease prevention. In rural areas, church health ministries may partner with local health departments or mobile clinics to bring medical services directly to their congregants.

For example, the Daniel Plan, a faith-based health program developed by Pastor Rick Warren, promotes healthy living through a combination of faith, food, fitness, and fellowship. The program encourages participants to make healthy lifestyle changes by incorporating spiritual practices, such as prayer and scripture reading, alongside practical health advice on diet and exercise.

Synagogue Health Outreach Programs

Synagogues have also been active in addressing health needs in their communities. Many synagogues run outreach programs that provide health services to underserved populations, including free medical clinics, mental health counseling, and food assistance. For example, B'nai B'rith International operates a network of senior housing facilities that provide affordable housing and healthcare services to low-income seniors, many of whom face significant health challenges.

Faith-Based Health Coalitions

In some communities, churches and synagogues have formed coalitions to address health disparities and advocate for health equity. These coalitions bring together faith leaders, healthcare providers, and community organizations to promote health and wellness on a broader scale. For example, the Faith-Based Health Equity Initiative in Chicago works to address health disparities in minority communities by providing health education, advocating for policy changes, and connecting residents with healthcare services.

CONCLUSION: BUILDING HEALTHIER COMMUNITIES THROUGH FAITH

The church and the synagogue have always been more than places of worship—they are centers of community life, support, and care. In small towns and inner cities, where health disparities and social challenges are often most acute, these institutions can play a pivotal role in promoting health and well-being. By providing health education, addressing mental health needs, reducing food insecurity, and advocating for health equity, religious institutions can contribute to making America healthy again.

Through faith-based health initiatives, churches and synagogues can leverage their unique position as trusted, respected institutions to address the social, physical, and spiritual determinants of health. With a focus on holistic care, these institutions can foster healthier, more resilient communities, ensuring that everyone has the opportunity to live a healthy and fulfilling life.

DR. CRANDALL'S AMERICA: The Role of Faith Communities in Health

Throughout my career, I have seen the power of faith-based organizations in shaping the health of their communities. Whether in small towns or inner cities, churches and synagogues have often filled critical gaps left by the healthcare system, providing education, support, and even medical care to those in need. At a time when healthcare is increasingly expensive and difficult to access, faith communities have stepped in to offer solutions that extend far beyond the walls of a hospital or doctor's office.

One of the most inspiring examples I have witnessed was in a small rural town where the local church started a wellness ministry. Many of the residents struggled with obesity, diabetes, and heart disease, but they lacked access to healthcare providers. The church began hosting free nutrition workshops, and walking groups and even invited medical professionals like myself to give talks on preventive care. I saw firsthand how these initiatives changed lives. One man, Greg, had been prediabetic for years but had never taken his condition seriously. After joining the church's health group, he lost 30 pounds, improved his diet, and reversed his diagnosis. "I never thought church would be the place that saved my health," he told me.

In inner cities, the role of faith organizations is just as vital, if not more so. I once worked with a synagogue in an urban neighborhood where access to healthy food was severely limited. The congregation took it upon themselves to start a community garden, providing fresh produce to families who otherwise relied on processed, unhealthy foods. They also organized weekly health screenings, where I and other medical volunteers checked blood pressure and glucose levels and offered guidance on managing chronic conditions. One elderly woman, Maria, who had never seen a doctor in years, discovered she had dangerously high blood pressure during one of these screenings. "I would have never known if I hadn't come here," she said. These efforts not only improved individual health outcomes but also fostered a sense of collective responsibility for well-being.

However, I have also seen the limitations of what faith-based organizations can do without greater systemic support. One church I worked with tried to establish a mental health program but struggled due to a lack of funding and professional resources. Many congregants were dealing with trauma, addiction, and anxiety, but there simply weren't enough therapists or counselors to meet the demand. A young man named David confided in me that he had been battling depression for years but felt ashamed to seek help. "I thought faith alone was supposed to fix me," he said. While faith can be a source of comfort, mental health requires comprehensive care—something that many religious organizations are not equipped to provide on their own.

Another challenge I have seen is the tension between faith and modern medicine. Some religious communities are hesitant about medical interventions, particularly vaccinations or certain treatments. I recall a case where a mother refused to vaccinate her children due to misinformation spread within her church. It took multiple conversations, backed by both medical evidence and input from trusted church leaders, to help her understand the importance of immunization. This experience reinforced for me that collaboration between faith leaders and healthcare professionals is essential to bridging gaps in medical knowledge and ensuring communities receive the best care possible.

Despite these challenges, I remain hopeful. I have seen churches partner with hospitals to provide mobile clinics, synagogues launch mental health awareness programs, and faith leaders use their platforms to promote healthier living. I have met pastors who advocate for better healthcare policies and rabbis who push for food justice in underserved areas. These efforts remind me that faith communities can be powerful allies in the fight for better health.

As a doctor, I have learned that healing is not just about medicine—it's about community, support, and access to the right resources. Churches and synagogues have always been places of refuge, and in many ways, they are becoming modern-day wellness centers. If we continue to strengthen the partnership between faith and healthcare, we can create a future where no one is left behind due to financial barriers, lack of access, or misinformation.

Faith has the power to heal, but it works best when combined with knowledge, compassion, and action. My hope is that more communities will embrace this potential, ensuring that every person—whether in a small town or an inner city—has the opportunity to live a healthier, fuller life.

R℞ Dr. Crandall's Prescription for the Role of Faith, Worship, and the Church in Making America's Small Towns and Big Cities Healthy Again

✔ **Leverage Faith-Based Communities for Health Support.** Engage with church and synagogue wellness programs that offer health education, fitness classes, and nutrition guidance.

✔ **Encourage Spiritual and Mental Well-Being.** Utilize faith-based teachings and support groups to reduce stress, manage anxiety, and foster emotional resilience.

✔ **Promote Healthy Eating in Religious Gatherings.** Advocate for nutritious meal options at community events, and encourage faith-based organizations to provide food assistance programs with whole, healthy foods.

✔ **Utilize Religious Networks for Healthcare Access.** Seek assistance from faith-based groups that provide free medical check-ups, screenings, and access to health resources for underserved communities.

✔ **Foster Interfaith Collaboration on Public Health Initiatives.** Support joint efforts among churches, synagogues, and community organizations to address issues like food insecurity, addiction recovery, and chronic disease prevention.

✔ **Encourage Walking Groups and Fitness Activities within Congregations.** Participate in faith-led movement initiatives like walking clubs, yoga sessions, or group exercise programs to promote physical health.

✔ **Educate on the Importance of Holistic Health.** Encourage faith leaders to incorporate health-focused messages into sermons, emphasizing the connection between spiritual well-being and physical wellness.

Resources

USA Churches
A searchable, nationwide directory of Christian churches across the United States; search by denomination, location, and other criteria (https://www.usachurches.org/).

Find a Synagogue
A locator to search for synagogues of any denomination in your area (https://www.shiva.com/learning-center/resources/find-a-synagogue?srsltid=AfmBOopwMl80oYqEGuPt_B4C-Lxp8oK1GAaQQvOpYZrxxIPeSKa04vlZ).

Catholic Charities USA
A directory to 168 centers of the nationwide Catholic Charities network offering a broad array of services to all people in need (https://www.catholiccharitiesusa.org/about-us/find-a-local-agency/).

B'nai B'rith International Center for Community Action
Community services for adults and children of the Jewish faith (https://www.bnaibrith.org/our-focus/humanitarian-aid/community -support/).

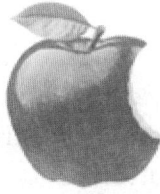

A BLUEPRINT FOR
A HEALTHIER AMERICA

DR. CRANDALL'S PRESCRIPTION

The journey through this book has explored the many facets of America's health crisis, offering a comprehensive roadmap for how individuals, communities, and governments can work together to create a healthier nation. Here are the key takeaways and solutions from each chapter, emphasizing the dual responsibility of personal actions and systemic changes needed to address the current challenges.

Key Actions for Individuals

- **Adopt a Healthy Diet (Food as Medicine).** Choose whole foods, reduce processed food intake, and focus on a plant-based, nutrient-rich diet. This approach can prevent and even reverse many chronic conditions.
- **Incorporate Regular Movement (Rethinking Exercise).** Make physical activity a daily habit, whether through walking, stretching, or functional exercises. Consistency, rather than intensity, is key to reaping the benefits of regular movement.

- **Prioritize Mental Health.** Practice mindfulness and meditation, and seek support when needed. Mental well-being is foundational to overall health, and addressing stress and anxiety can lead to better physical health outcomes.
- **Engage in Preventive Healthcare.** Regular check-ups and screenings are vital for early detection and prevention of disease. Take charge of your health by staying informed and proactive about your healthcare needs.
- **Build Strong Social Connections.** Strengthen ties with family, friends, and community groups. Social support plays a crucial role in mental and physical health, reducing the risk of isolation and promoting resilience.
- **Advocate for Personal Health Rights.** Stay informed about health policies, and advocate for transparent, patient-centered healthcare. Use your voice to support better access to healthcare and policies that prioritize preventive care.

Key Actions for Government and Communities

- **Reform Healthcare Policy for Prevention.** Shift focus from reactive treatment to preventive care. Policies should prioritize early interventions, lifestyle education, and access to primary care, reducing the burden of chronic diseases.
- **Promote Access to Healthy Food.** Implement policies that make nutritious foods more affordable and accessible, particularly in food deserts. Support local farming, improve food labeling, and incentivize healthier food options in schools and public institutions.
- **Invest in Urban Planning for Active Living.** Design walkable cities with accessible green spaces, bike lanes, and safe recreational areas. By creating environments that encourage physical activity, communities can foster healthier lifestyles.

- **Address Mental Health at the Policy Level.** Increase funding for mental health services, and integrate mental health care into primary care settings. Public awareness campaigns can help reduce stigma and encourage people to seek the help they need.
- **Combat Health Misinformation.** Launch educational campaigns to provide accurate, evidence-based information on health topics, including the risks and benefits of vaccinations. Support health literacy programs to help the public make informed decisions.
- **Support Health Equity Initiatives.** Tackle systemic health disparities by improving access to quality healthcare, nutritious food, and safe environments, especially in underserved communities. Policies should address the social determinants of health to ensure fair opportunities for all.
- **Promote Sustainable Health Practices.** Implement environmental policies that reduce pollution and support sustainable farming. A focus on eco-health initiatives can improve public health and protect the planet for future generations.

Vision for a Healthier Future

The path to making America healthy again requires a holistic approach that integrates individual responsibility with comprehensive policy changes. By embracing the principles of preventive care, prioritizing mental well-being, and promoting equity in health access, we can lay the foundation for a thriving, resilient nation.

A healthier America is not only possible—it is essential for the well-being of future generations. By taking action now, at both the personal and policy levels, we can create a society where every individual has the opportunity to live a long, healthy, and fulfilling life. Let this book be a call to action for everyone: to take steps today toward a healthier tomorrow and to work collectively toward building a nation that values health as its greatest wealth.

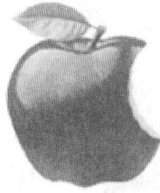

ACKNOWLEDGMENTS

First and foremost, to my wife Deborah—you've been my rock, my sounding board, and my constant advocate. Your devotion to our family and your tireless work as a home health advocate inspire me every single day. This book wouldn't exist without your love and encouragement.

To Chris Ruddy at NewsMax Media—I'll never forget that conversation over fifteen years ago when you took a chance on me and encouraged me to write a medical newsletter. That opportunity put me on a path I could never have imagined, and I remain deeply grateful for your faith in me.

To Charlotte Libov, who has been my steady hand and sharp eye for so many years—thank you for your gentle but firm edits, your knack for making my words shine, and your patience through countless drafts. You've made me a better writer and a better communicator.

And to Dr. Peter Fielding and Dr. Larry Cohen at Yale University School of Medicine—your belief in me as both a clinician and a research scientist gave me the confidence to chase ideas that mattered. Your past mentorship and encouragement have left a lasting mark not only on my career, but also on me as a person.

To all of you—you've each shaped this journey in your own special way. This book is as much yours as it is mine, and I'm forever grateful.

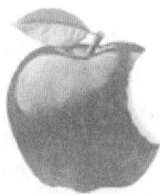

INDEX

ABOUT THE AUTHOR

Renowned Cardiologist, Author, and Global Health Advocate

Dr. Chauncey Crandall is widely regarded as one of the nation's foremost cardiologists, known for his pioneering work in both interventional cardiology and concierge medicine. Over a career spanning decades, he has earned a reputation for excellence in patient care, advanced cardiovascular research, and shown a commitment to bringing high-quality medical care to people worldwide.

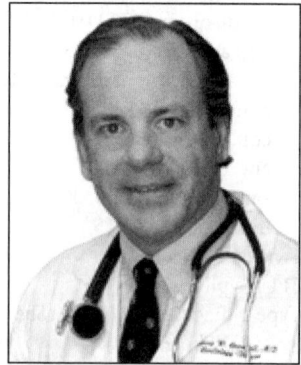

Distinguished Training and Medical Background

Currently based in Palm Beach, Florida, Dr. Crandall's medical journey began with rigorous academic and clinical training at some of the world's most respected institutions. He studied at Yale University and Harvard University, followed by prestigious fellowships at Beth Israel Hospital and the Medical College of Virginia. His broad training across internal medicine and cardiology equipped him with the knowledge and skills to address even the most complex medical conditions.

In the past, Dr. Crandall played a pivotal role in establishing Duke University's Florida Interventional Cardiology Program, bringing cutting-edge techniques and innovations in cardiovascular care to patients in the region. Throughout his career, he has also been affiliated with, and served in leadership roles at, several leading medical centers in Palm Beach, Florida and beyond.

Professional Achievements

Dr. Crandall's career is defined by measurable accomplishments:

- 40,000+ medical procedures performed, including high-risk cardiac interventions.
- 2,000+ publications contributing to the global body of cardiology and medical care and research.
- A monthly medical newsletter delivered to hundreds of thousands of subscribers worldwide since 2010, offering practical heart-health advice and the latest medical insights.
- An unwavering focus on patient-centered care, combining advanced evidence-based medicine with personalized treatment strategies.

Author, Educator, and Public Speaker

Beyond the operating room and clinic, Dr. Crandall is an influential voice in public health education. He is the best-selling author of books including *The Simple Heart Cure*, a widely praised guide to preventing and reversing heart disease, and *Touching Heaven*, an inspiring memoir blending his medical career with personal experiences of faith and hope.

As a sought-after speaker, he has addressed professional audiences, faith-based gatherings, and community health events around the world, sharing both his expertise and his deeply human approach to medicine. His talks emphasize prevention, lifestyle transformation, and the profound connection between physical and spiritual well-being.

Commitment to Global Health

Dr. Crandall's mission extends far beyond his local practice. He has traveled internationally to perform medical missions, conduct research, and train other physicians in developing nations. His humanitarian work reflects his belief that quality healthcare is a universal right, and his goal is to make life-saving medicine accessible wherever it is needed most.

Vision and Philosophy of Care

At the core of Dr. Crandall's approach to medicine is the conviction that healing involves more than just technology and science— it requires compassion, listening, and treating patients as whole individuals. He blends state-of-the-art cardiology and internal medicine with a personal, private-level service model, ensuring that each patient receives attentive, unhurried, and comprehensive care.

To contact Dr. Crandall:

> Dr. Chauncey Crandall
> c/o Chadwick Foundation
> P.O. Box 3046
> Palm Beach, FL 33480

Vist the author at ChaunceyCrandall.com.

To learn more, go to Dr. Chauncey Crandall's Heart Health Report for a Symptom, Drug & Stress Free Life at DrCrandall.Newsmax.com.